MODERN VETERINARY PRACTICE MANAGEMENT

ANIMAL SCIENCE, ISSUES AND PROFESSIONS

Additional books in this series can be found on Nova's website
under the Series tab.

Additional e-books in this series can be found on Nova's website
under the e-book tab.

ANIMAL SCIENCE, ISSUES AND PROFESSIONS

MODERN VETERINARY PRACTICE MANAGEMENT

MARGIT GABRIELE MULLER

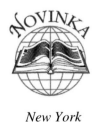

New York

Library of Congress Cataloging-in-Publication Data

Modern veterinary practice management / editor, Margit Gabriele Muller.
    p. ; cm.
 Includes bibliographical references and index.
 ISBN: 978-1-62808-858-8 (softcover)
 I. Muller, Margit Gabriele.
 [DNLM: 1. Practice Management--organization & administration. 2. Veterinary Medicine--organization & administration. 3. Hospitals, Animal. SF 756.4]
  636.089--dc23
                           2011042415

Published by Nova Science Publishers, Inc. † New York

CONTENTS

PREFACE

The book "Modern Veterinary Practice Management" by Dr. Margit Gabriele Muller represents a comprehensive, well-structured reference book on veterinary practice management not to be missed, if one starts a new veterinary entity or if one is looking to improve the business of an existing one of any size or type. The book contains a lot of advice on running the veterinary practice smoothly, efficiently and successfully by taking its financial performance to the maximum benefit into account without compromising on excellent veterinary medical service for the clients. It transforms the modern business management knowledge into an easy step-by-step improvement approach for the everyday veterinary practice work.

Its novel synthesis between practical everyday application and theoretical business management background information provides its audience with an insight into the workings of veterinary practices, clinics and hospitals based on many years of experience as a veterinarian and business woman. The reference book has been written for veterinarians, veterinary practice managers, veterinary students as well as veterinary technicians, practice administrators and practice associates.

"Modern Veterinary Practice Management" covers all relevant topics ranging from changes in veterinary practice management, operations management, finances and budgeting, marketing, administration, human resources and IT. It is illustrated with tables and diagrams to facilitate an easier understanding of topics, which may be regarded as remote but will prove crucial to the entity's survival, i.e. finances, leadership or the quest for excellence.

Written by Dr. med. vet. Margit Gabriele Muller MBA, managerial and veterinary Director of the Abu Dhabi Falcon Hospital, the world largest veterinary hospital specialized on the treatment of birds of prey, this outstanding book draws on her long personal day to day experience in growing the entity from a small practice-sized clinic to its world-class status today. In her dual role as the experienced hospital manager and world-wide renowned veterinary specialist in avian medicine Dr. Muller not only understands the specific requirements of modern veterinary practices but has implemented the tools described in the reference book in her everyday work at the Abu Dhabi Falcon Hospital and makes her broad experience available for you.

FOREWORD

The idea for this book was developed during my studies of Master of Business Administration at the University of Strathclyde, Glasgow, which was a far cry from knowledge obtained during my veterinary studies. The classical veterinary education revolves around the anatomy, physiology, diseases and their treatment of the bovine, avian, equine, swine species and the assorted small animals. At that stage, none of my fellow students nor myself pictured us as small business entrepreneurs other than in the medical running of a veterinary practice or clinic. Anything related to administration, finance, accounting or let alone marketing, controlling operations and supply-chain management were issues not directly related to the future we all envisioned. Naturally, we all lacked the skills in the field of veterinary practice management.

Against this educational background, I came a long way from being a pure veterinary surgeon to becoming a veterinary surgeon cum businesswoman. During my ten years of practicing veterinary medicine in the very specialized environment of the Abu Dhabi Falcon Hospital it became quite clear that caring for and curing animals will not be sufficient to ensure the survival of the then small avian clinic. After my promotion to being the director of this unique hospital for falcons the daily responsibilities expanded very quickly from veterinary treatment to managing staff, ensuring medical supply, increasing the customer base, strategically realign the business model to the customer demand and beyond. During my 10 years in Abu Dhabi, my excellent and motivated team and I developed the previously small clinic to the largest falcon hospital worldwide by employing reasonable methods of business administration and management on a step by step basis.

During this time, I learned to appreciate the reasoning of both the veterinary profession in its medical care, innovation and scientific logic but also the tools and laws of the business world which cannot be ignored, if a veterinary practice shall survive. It is the reasonable synthesis of both, which eventually leads to profound business success and a medical reputation of excellence.

My sincerest gratitude goes to H.E. Mohammed Al Bowardi, who entrusted me the Abu Dhabi Falcon Hospital both in the role as a veterinarian and business manager to live up to the vision of H.H. The Late Sheikh Zayed bin Sultan Al Nahyan to provide public veterinary treatment to the falcons of the falconers of the Abu Dhabi emirate. His great continuous support and vision inspired and still inspires my team and me to live up to the expectation of all falconers to receive the best medical care and services possible.

I would like to thank H.E. Majid Al Mansouri, who provided me with the support and freedom to lead independently the Abu Dhabi Falcon Hospital on the path of tremendous growth, expansion and diversification to become the largest hospital world-wide specialized in the treatment of these magnificent birds of prey.

The experiences in veterinary practice/hospital management are not restricted to the management of an avian veterinary hospital. They are valid for any veterinary entity no matter how large or small and were tested against the theories in business administration during my MBA studies. During that time, I have received great support from Mr. Amer Abu Aabed with whom I wrote many assignments and the master thesis during our MBA time. We challenged ourselves to find new solutions and to regard processes from a different point of view in order to improve our work at the Abu Dhabi Falcon Hospital. I am highly grateful to Mr. Amer Abu Aabed as he encouraged me to realize my dream to write this book on veterinary practice management and Mr. Kishore Kumar whose IT know-how helped greatly for this book.

A very big thank you goes to all of my excellent team at the Abu Dhabi Falcon Hospital without whom the success of the Abu Dhabi Hospital would never been achievable and whose personalities, knowledge and professionalism are a joy to work with.

My sincerest and very special thanks go to my family, my father Helmut, my mother Hertha and my sister Andrea. Their support and encouragement during my years of studies and veterinary work has been a great stronghold and encouragement for me, especially during difficult times. My parents laid the foundation for me to become the person I am today. Their values formed my personality and provided me with an open mind and my love of animals. Moreover, I am most grateful to my sister Andrea for her great support and for reviewing this manuscript despite her time constraints.

Dr. med. vet. Margit Gabriele Muller MBA, MRCVS
Abu Dhabi, United Arab Emirates
September 2011

LIST OF ABBREVIATIONS

AAHA	American Animal Hospital Association
Amp	Ampoule
AP	Approve
B2B	Business-to-Business
B2C	Business-to-Customer
BC	Biochemistry
BEP	Break-even point
BSC	Balanced Scorecard
C2B	Customer-to-Business
C2C	Customer-to-Customer
CNS	Central nervous system
CPA	Certified Public Accountant
CT	Computed tomography
CV	Curriculum vitae
DR	Disaster recovery
DVM	Doctor of Veterinary Medicine
e.g.	"exempli gratia' (Latin), for example
EQ	Emotional quotient
etc.	Etcetera
FM	Finance Manager
FTE	Full time equivalent
g	Gram
G2C	Government-to-Citizen
Hb	Hemoglobin
Hct	Hematocrit
HN	Head Nurse
HRM	Human Resources Manager
HV	Head Veterinarian
i.e.	"id est" (Latin), that is/it is/in other words
IQ	Intelligence quotient
ISO	International Organization for Standardization
KPI	Key performance indicator
MBA	Master of Business Administration

mg	Milligram
ml	Milliliter
MRSA	Methicillin-resistant *Staphylococcus aureus*
no.	Number
NPV	Net Present Value
OHSAS	Occupational Health and Safety Assessment Series
pcs	Pieces
PM	Performance Management
PM	Practice Manager
PMS	Performance Management System
PO	Practice owner
PP	Performance Prism
PP	payback period
Q	Quarter
RBC	Red blood cell count
RC	Recommend
RCVS	Royal College of Veterinary Surgeons
RI	Residual income
RIDF	Radio-frequency identification tags
ROCE	Return on Capital Employed
ROE	Return on Equity
ROSF	Return on Shareholders' Funds
RV	Review
SCM	Supply Chain Management
SFO	Strategy-focused organization
SME	small and medium-sized enterprises
SPU	Sales revenue per unit
SWOT	Strengths, weaknesses, opportunities, threats
tbl	Tablet
TFC	Total fixed costs
UK	United Kingdom
USA	United States of America
USP	Unique selling proposition / point
V	Veterinarian
VAT	Value Added Tax
VCU	Variable costs per unit
VOIP	Voice over IP
vs.	Versus
WBC	White blood cell count

Chapter 1

INTRODUCTION

ABSTRACT

During the past decades, veterinary medicine has grown beyond its original purpose of treating animals, as it has turned from the operating theatre into small and medium-sized businesses providing veterinary services. This current trend in veterinary medicine demands a much higher degree of detailed, business-oriented knowledge from veterinarians and practice owners due to the animal owner requesting a much larger variety of services nowadays. In contrast to the traditional approach of curing animals in one's own practice by purchasing a few instruments, tables and starting in rented or one's own premises by often taking over an established practice, today a business idea for the new veterinary practice has to be formulated before setting up a veterinary practice. Following the clear business idea, major business-related issues in the form of a well-thought and well-structured business plan have to be addressed. Furthermore, sufficient knowledge of financial, administrative and operation management are mandatory for a successful veterinary practice and will be required by any financial institution financing the undertaking.

1.1. INTRODUCTION

The veterinary world has undergone tremendous changes in the past decades. The average modern veterinary practice is not any longer an isolated small business focused on the performance of veterinary medicine with some accounting for tax purposes at the end of the year and great deal of altruism anymore, but reinvented itself as a small enterprise combining increasingly high-value veterinary medical services with an up-to-date management approach. The current trends in veterinary medicine have catapulted veterinarians in an ever increasing competitive and comprehensive business world, something they had not been used to, and they were not educated for. New services like pet behavior, homeopathic treatment, pet husbandry and grooming services are now part of the products and services requested by customers [3]. Often having started in the United States and being transferred to Europe as 'state of the art' through scientific and popular media, this development needs to be taken seriously into consideration for a successful veterinary practice. This book intends to highlight and discuss models of a modular veterinary practice with modern management features that may assist to meet both, these new requirements as well as the ever-changing needs of customers. Although veterinarians do not usually regard themselves as business persons or managers, they may have to adapt their perception of their position and practices to survive and succeed in an increasingly challenging and competitive veterinary world [3].

1.2. Major Factors for Setting up a Veterinary Practice

Veterinary practices are usually defined as small or even very small enterprises as part of the economic categorization 'small and medium-sized enterprises (SME)' by employing up to 20 staff members [2]. Small enterprises do not only form the large majority of businesses, but they are also the vital drivers of the economy [5]. The main reason for failures of SMEs applies to the failure of veterinary practices as well, namely poor management knowledge [1, 2, 3]. Both, veterinary practices and SMEs require careful medium-term planning to avoid pitfalls in the set up phase.

Following the recent developments and trends in the veterinary world, the traditional single service practice offering veterinary treatment only has been in many cases taken over by more comprehensive practice models. Clients would be willing to pay a small annual fee for a membership card offering promotions, information, incentives, gift vouchers for such a one-stop shop veterinary practice [3]. However, the newly opened veterinary practice will have to offer all reasonable veterinary treatments like surgery, ultrasound and X-ray diagnosis. Yet, in the 21st century, these medical services are expected to be upgraded by specific offers like pet shops, home delivery, boarding facilities, "pet-sitting" and wellness/alternative and specialist medicine. The scope of the practice always entirely depends on its specialization as e.g. a referral practice for dentistry requires other premises, equipment, instruments and business strategies than a general practice [3].

One of the most important factors to ensure the success of the newly established veterinary practice is a thorough understanding of one's competitor situation. Competitor worksheets may be of great assistance in evaluating one's competing veterinarians (for details, please refer to chapter 3). Moreover, it might lead to the understanding and identifying of a specialized niche market focusing on certain species (e.g. birds, reptiles) or services (e.g. dentistry, ophthalmology, dermatology). The consumer potential and income situation in this area is another key to success [3].

Clear analysis of the market situation and potential customer is essential for the survival of the new business venture [2, 4]. New business owners need to be able to understand and be familiar with the most important basic financial terms, key performance indicators (KPI) like ratios [2] as well as control mechanisms to see early-warning signs in time if the business does not develop as expected [3]. Financial management as well as accounting skills are often not enough appreciated by veterinarians, which might lead to major problems afterwards. People management and training are another area, which is often underestimated, too.

One of the most important first activities when setting up a new veterinary practice is a good well-thought detailed and well-structured business plan. This plan should include the explanation of the main business idea, information of the owner, intended legal set up, business area, market study and competitors as well as a profound financial planning [6] not only for the next few months but also with a medium-term outlook.

The first crucial factor for success is the choice of the location for the newly established practice. In this context, the number of pets in the area, a critical look at the parking situation for clients, infrastructure and rents [7] are to be taken into account. Important features to support modern veterinary practices are premises layout, workflow plans and professional work environment. The well-designed layout of the premises according to smooth and efficient workflow enables fast and productive work with reduced waiting times for the customers. The professionally structured workplace leads to quality work and avoids unnecessary time loss thus resulting in higher overall efficiency and greater staff and customer satisfaction [3].

The current trends in veterinary medicine and the higher competitive business environments force veterinarians to change. Change in a traditionally more conservative profession means not only acquiring more sound business knowledge, but also finding a sustainable competitive advantage compared to the other veterinary practices. This may be achieved by offering new additional services like high-tech diagnostic equipment and treatment, wellness/alternative medicine in a soothing environment, dog behavior and obedience training courses as well as pet shops integrated in the veterinary practices. These additional services of a contemporary, state-of-the-art veterinary practice will form an enhancement of the customer's and pet's lifestyle through the hassle-free, time saving one-stop-shop concept. Excellent quality as well as fast and efficient delivery of the services on offer will greatly assist in building up a loyal, long-term customer base [3].

1.3. CONCLUSION

The topic of modern veterinary practice management may be interesting, especially for all veterinary practitioners working in any kind of practice or veterinary clinic as scientific thinking usually differs greatly from the business mindset. This may broaden one's horizon by creating a new world of experiences by merging a newly acquired deeper understanding of business issues with the inquisitive scientific background. In this light, scientific and business thinking becomes a highly comprehensive and wide ranging. By combining these two apparently contradictory fields of expertise today's veterinary practitioners would be well equipped to successfully manage all issues arising in the day to day business of a veterinary enterprise with the maximum benefit for a successful veterinary practice.

This book may provide veterinary practitioners with a structured approach to explore veterinary practice concepts from a business point of view and apply modern business knowledge in a simplified form into their own veterinary practice.

REFERENCES

[1]   Brown, J.P. and Silverman, J.D. (1999). The current and future market for veterinarians and veterinary medical services in the United States. *JAVMA*, Vol. 215, No. 2, July 15. pp. 161-183.

[2] Megginson, W.L., Byrd, M.J. and Megginson, L.C. (2000). *Small business management: An entrepreneur's guidebook.* 3rd ed. McGraw-Hill. Boston, Madrid, Toronto.

[3] Müller, M.G. and Abu Aabed, A. (2007). *Guidelines for setting up a small and medium size enterprise.* MBA Thesis, University of Strathclyde. Graduate School of Business. Glasgow.

[4] Ryan, J.D. and Hiduke, G.P. (2006). *Small business: an entrepreneur's business plan.* 7th ed. Thompson South-Western. Ohio.

[5] The Entrepreneur Magazine (1999). *Small business advisor.* 2nd ed. John Entrepreneur Media Inc. Wiley&Sons. New York, Chichester, Weinheim, Brisbane, Singapore, Toronto.

[6] Vetline (2003). Erfolg mit schlüssigem Business Plan. March 31st. http://www.vetline.de/vetservices/praxismanager/geld_und_recht/business-plan_erfolg .htm (Accessed on October 11th, 2006)

[7] Vetline (2006). Quo vadis, Tierarztpraxis? July 9th. http://www.vetline.de/ vetservices/praxismanager/geld_und_recht/standortanalyse_tierarztpraxis.htm(Accessed on October 11th, 2006).

Chapter 2

CURRENT TRENDS IN VETERINARY PRACTICES

ABSTRACT

Veterinary practices have changed tremendously over the past years due to a multitude of factors. One major trend is the already mentioned integration of new services like pet husbandry, grooming, wellness and alternative medicines like homeopathy and acupuncture. Another important trend to watch is the rising number of veterinary specializations in species, diagnostic services and veterinary treatments. Pet ownership is shifting from traditional pets to exotic pets. From the legal and business point of view, the form of establishment currently is undergoing a major change opening up sole proprietorship and partnership to allowing limited liabilities companies to be established in an increasing number of countries. Major changes in the gender ratio are meanwhile taking place with the majority of female veterinary medicine students worldwide. However, this does not reflect as a positive impact on the salary differences among male and female veterinarians and the imbalance among mostly male veterinary practice owners and female veterinary assistants.

2.1. INTRODUCTION

In the 1950s, the picture of the good old Dr. James Herriot taking care of the large animal population was the famous idol that veterinarian students worldwide would like to mirror in their professional life and that has motivated many veterinary student generations to take up this profession.

Over the last decades, this picture has changed tremendously as the previously dominant large animal practices have considerably disappeared in favor of small animal or combined large and small animal practices [22]. However, in the past 10 years new trends have come up in veterinary medicine, as pet owners tend to emotionalize their pets increasingly leading pet owners to expect the same medical services for their pets, as they would expect to receive as human beings [31].

This behavioral change in customer demand has led to the trend setting inclusion of services like pet husbandry and grooming, behavior therapy, massage and homeopathy into the spectrum of veterinary services [26, 31]. Well-known in humans, wellness has found its way into veterinary medicine in various areas like equine medicine and wellness for horses. These latest developments now include alternative medicine like acupuncture, chiropractic and homeopathy [21]. Homeopathic and Bach's flower treatment is used for many different diseases in small animals [15] as well as in birds [13, 19, 27]. Pets [18], large animals and birds are also treated with acupuncture [22, 27].

In order to offer a broader choice for the clients, practices have placed themselves in direct competition to traditional dog and cat grooming salons as well as classical pet shops.

The convenient one-stop-for-all strategy combined with the aura of medical expertise seems to pay off and add a major competitive advantage. Relatively new areas of medical services are professional nutrition consultations for pets and dog behavior consultations by veterinary professionals. In addition, certain practices either have expanded their laboratory facilities or restricted themselves to provide exclusively advanced laboratory services for patients and other veterinary practices alike.

2.2. TRENDS IN VETERINARY SERVICES AND SPECIALIZATION

In Europe, the current trend leads a rising number of small animal practices, which have outgrown and in some areas substituted the large animal practices by far [21]. However, this development directly leads to a higher competition in the small animal practice sector [22]. Sole large animal practices are on the decline as the number of large animals is dwindling and the areas of professional agricultural farming are reducing fast [23].

Mirroring the development in human medical clinics, more and more veterinarian practitioners decide to set up exclusive referral clinics for special disciplines like surgery, dermatology, cardiology or specialized visual diagnostic centers for ultra-sound, C-bow technology and/or computed tomography as the latest trend among predominately small animal practices.

A very modern development follows the increase in keeping exotic pets by opening of practices solely specialized in one species only i.e. in felines or exotic animal species like reptiles or birds [21, 22].

This increasing number of recognized veterinary specializations can be also observed in the increased variety of veterinary specialization courses offered and the rising number of certified veterinary experts acquiring specialized diplomas:

Table 2.1. Development of recognized veterinary specialty diplomates in USA from 2006 to 2009 [1, 2, 3, 4]

Year	Number of diplomates
2006	8,510
2007	8,885
2008	9,305
2009	9,826

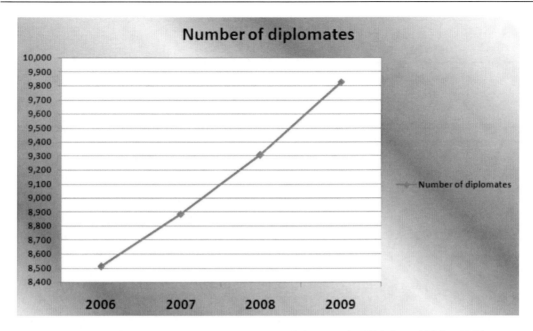

Figure 2.1. Numbers of recognized veterinary specialty diplomates in USA from 2006 to 2009 [1, 2, 3, 4].

2.3. TRENDS IN PETS OWNERSHIP

The patient clientele of small animal practices has undergone a significant change since the 1990s. Until twenty years ago, the majority of pets consisted of dogs and cats and the odd budgie or rabbit. Since that time, an increasing number of pet owners has switched to birds, fish, reptiles and small rodents like rabbits, turtles or hamsters and all sorts of exotic creatures, which were available before mostly to the rather rich and eccentric pet owners. Due to an increasing 'humanization' of pets, the number of dogs and cats slightly rose during the past years more often than not substituting human partners for lonely pet owners.

Table 2.2. Development of pet ownership in USA 2001 compared to 2007 [5, 6]

	Dogs 2001	Dogs 2007	Cats 2001	Cats 2007	Birds 2001	Birds 2007	Horses 2001	Horses 2007
% of households owning	36.1 %	37.2 %	31.6 %	32.4 %	4.6 %	3.9 %	1.7 %	1.8 %
Numbers of households owning	37,900 Mio	43,021 Mio	33,186 Mio	37,460 Mio	4,818 Mio	4,453 Mio	1,751 Mio	2,087 Mio
Average number per household	1.6	1.7	2.1	2.2	2.1	2.5	2.9	3.5

In UK, a survey of the Royal College of Veterinary Surgeons [24] displays a quite similar development of pet ownership.

Table 2.3. Development of pet ownership in UK 2001, 2006, 2010 and predicted 2015 in % [24]

	2001 in %	2006 in %	2010 in %	2015 (2010 predicted) in %
Dogs	33.8	33.5	35.7	33.11
Cats	27.6	29.1	29.1	28.88
Birds	1	1.1	1.02	0.96
Horses	9.2	9.2	9.98	10.98
Exotics	0.6	0.6	0.75	0.87
Cattle	10.6	8.2	7.2	7.3

In some veterinary practices, the numbers of small rodent and small mammal patients form up to 12 % of the total patient number with rising tendency [23]. A major increase in fish, turtles, snakes, lizards and other birds can be observed in USA from 2001 to 2007.

Table 2.4. Development of exotic pets in USA 2001 compared to 2007 [5, 6]

Animal species	Households 2001 (in 1,000)	Households 2007 (in 1,000)	Population 2001 (in 1,000)	Population 2007 (in 1,000)
Fish	6,396	9,036	49,251	75,898
Ferrets	472	505	991	1,060
Rabbits	1,783	1,870	4,813	6,171
Hamsters	734	826	881	1,239
Guinea pigs	524	628	629	1,004
Gerbils	168	187	319	431
Other rodents	315	452	786	949
Turtles	629	1,106	1,070	1,991
Snakes	315	390	661	586
Lizards	419	719	545	1,078
Other reptiles	315	69	598	199
Other birds	315	464	2,894	4,966
Livestock	524	728	2,936	10,995
All others	839	1,182	2,013	3,664

2.4. TRENDS IN PET OWNER DEMOGRAPHICS

Although the number of veterinary visits for dogs and cats per household showed a mild decline in the United States of America from 2001 to 2007, the average veterinary expenditure per household rose for all animal species. This trend can be regarded as a very positive one for the veterinarians as dog owners are more likely to spend more money on an annual basis on their pets than cat owners. However, apart from dogs' owners, the veterinary expenditure per animal in households has remained stable or declined over the past years [5, 6]. The impact of the global recession in 2009 and 2010 on veterinary expenditures has not been fully recorded statistically but is expected to affect negatively this trend at least in certain countries most hit by the crises.

Table 2.5. Development of pet owners' expenditure in USA 2001 compared to 2007 [5, 6]

	Dogs 2001	Dogs 2007	Cats 2001	Cats 2007	Birds 2001	Birds 2007	Horses 2001	Horses 2007
Veterinary visits per household per year (mean)	2.7	2.6	1.8	1.7	0.3	0.3	2.1	2.2
Veterinary expenditure per household per year (mean)	$ 261	$ 356	$ 160	$ 190	$ 18	$ 25	$ 263	$ 360
Veterinary expenditure per animal (mean)	$ 179	$ 200	$ 85	$ 81	$ 9	$ 9	$ 112	$ 92

2.5. TRENDS AND IMPLICATIONS OF IMBALANCED RATIO FEMALE-MALE VETERINARIANS

Over the last years, female students have been taking the lead studying veterinary medicine. Already in 1999, in Germany 87.74% of veterinary students were female with rising tendency [30]. In the USA, female students represented approximately 70% of all veterinary students in 1999. They are expected to reach 78% in 2015 [11]. Despite this high number, female veterinarians in USA pose only approximately half of practicing veterinarians. However, their number was rising constantly over the past years whereas the number of male veterinarians remained stable. Female graduates are in general younger than their male counterparts with 71% of female veterinary surgeons below the age of 40 years [24]. However, due to parental leave and child care 13% of these female surgeons take career breaks requiring cover by more flexible work arrangements or more staff involved to cover the work load [24]. Moreover, female veterinary surgeons as employees work less than 40 hours per week twice more than females and male practice owners, and their income is 30% lower compared to their male counterparts. One reason lies in the fact of female veterinarians tend to concentrate more on opening their small clinic in a town or suburb [14].

Another reason for this discrepancy in working hours might be part-time work, children's care and fewer obligations in the veterinary practice as many administrative duties are traditionally performed by the practice owner. The part-time work of up to 75% female veterinarians in the UK leads to an extra need of 40% fresh graduates [26].

Table 2.6. Development of male and female veterinarians in USA from 2006 to 2009 [7, 8, 9, 10]

Year	Male	Female	Total
2006	43,112	38,356	81,356
2007	43,196	40,534	83,730
2008	43,287	42,690	85,977
2009	43,196	44,802	87,998

Table 2.7. Development of positions in veterinary practice in UK 2002 compared to 2006 [25]

	2002 Total in %	2006 Total in %	2006 Male in %	2006 Female in %
Sole principal	14	11	17	5
Partner/director of limited Company	-	10	16	4
Salaried partner	-	2	2	1
Partner	-	16	25	7
Total partner	24	28	43	12
Full-time assistant	43	40	28	52
Part-time assistant	11	11	3	20
Consultant	-	1	2	1
Locum	9	6	5	8
Other	-	2	1	2

Another major discrepancy between male and female veterinarians can be found in their hierarchical position in veterinary practices. Male veterinarians mainly hold senior positions while almost ¾ of females are employed as full-time or part-time assistants [25].

In Germany, the situation is relatively similar. Female veterinarians represent a much larger portion of veterinary practice assistants representing almost ¾ of all employed assistants [20].

2.6. TRENDS OF THE INCOME SITUATION OF VETERINARIANS

Currently, the supply of veterinarians exceeds the demand of veterinarians most markedly in the USA, which is by far the largest market for veterinarians. Until 2008, forecasts did predict a similar picture hence creating a major pressure on the income and prices for veterinary services due to veterinary oversupply. From 2008 to 2014, the supply and demand was indicated to balance as the consequence resulting in a more relaxed situation on the service price and income structure [11]. Newer data that may confirm or contradict these predictions are not yet ready available.

Regarding the real income situation, major differences have become obvious regarding the status of the veterinarians compared to owners and associates of veterinary practices not only in the USA but also in European countries [22]. Compared to other medical disciplines, veterinarians were ranking last with a mean income of US$ 57,130 compared to physicians and surgeons with US$ 102,000 ranking first in 1998 [14].

The average annual salary of veterinarians in USA has increased to US$79,050 in 2008 whereas the salary of veterinarians employed in the Federal Government is higher with an average $93,398 in 2009 [12]. In UK, the average basic salary for full-time veterinarians is just below £49,000, which is almost 1/3 up to ½ less than the yearly salaries of human doctors [25].

This should be kept in mind when deciding to start a veterinary business [22]. Moreover, major differences in the income situation between male and female veterinarians as self-employed practice can be observed in various countries.

Table 2.8. Income imbalance of male and female veterinarians in Germany in 2001 and 2004 (excluding practice assistants) [16, 17]

Year	Total	Male Veterinarians (in Euro)	Females veterinarians (in Euro)
1998	38,835		
2001	45,138	53,076	26,007
2004	47,483	56,335	28,927

The income situation of veterinarians that are employed as full-time or part-time veterinary practice assistants is much worse. Female veterinary practice assistants earn an average monthly salary of 2,400 euros before tax, which is 550 euros less than their male counterparts [20].

2.7. TRENDS IN THE VETERINARY BUSINESS MANAGEMENT AND REASONS FOR FAILURE

While in the veterinary curricula worldwide medical subjects cover approximately 99% of the curricula, courses in business and economics usually count only for 1%. By contrast, in the real work situation 85% of the veterinarian's time is spent on business and communication matters, and only approx. 15% on the actual veterinary medical work. This indicates a considerable lack of both income and business management knowledge by veterinary profession compared to other medical professions [22, 29].

Most small businesses fail not necessarily due to professional incompetence, but due to lack of management knowledge and skills [11]. Small businesses in the USA are unsuccessful as they lack capital (48%) and often manage their businesses inadequately due to 23% missing business knowledge, 19% poor management, 15% insufficient planning and 15% inexperience [21]. These special problems more often than not may result in reduced profitability and growth, leading to financial problems and subsequently closure of the business [21, 22].

When analyzed closely there does not seem to exist a major difference between the failure of small businesses and that of veterinary practices. Both can be traced usually to inadequate management: "Thirty-eight percent of the practice owners … said they had observed practice failures. The 5 most frequently mentioned reasons for practice failures are insufficient client base (39%), new competition (25%), poor client management (24%), unsatisfactory office management (22%), and lacking communication skills (20%)." [11, p.180, 22]. Other reasons for failure seem to be inadequate marketing activities, excessively high costs, deficient understanding of customer needs, insufficient own capital and cash flow as well as not sufficiently high turnover [22, 30].

These discrepancies have led to major studies by KPMG and Brakke Consulting to obtain a deeper insight in the market and income situation of veterinarians [11, 14]. According to the KPMG study, the delivery of veterinary services and animal care is performed "through a highly fragmented and inefficient system" [11, p.162]. Although there is a good market for veterinarians in nontraditional and non private areas, they often "lack some of the skills and aptitudes that result in economic success" [11, p.162]. This is also supported by the fact that general business best practice like benchmarking is a relatively unknown phenomenon in the veterinary field [28].

2.8. CONCLUSION

Significant trends in veterinary medicine cover changes in pet ownership, gender distribution and income development. Hereby, the continuous reduction in large animal ownership shifted to a similarly continuous rise in small animals' ownership, especially in pets. A relatively unique feature in the scientific field is the high number of female students leading to the subsequent rise of female veterinary practitioners. However, the impact of this new female veterinary force has not yet found its way into veterinary practice ownership as female veterinarians mainly are employed as assistant veterinarians. Mirroring the development in human medicine, the specialization of veterinarians and the related increase in board certifications can be classified as a new trend as well. This leads to a much more refined quality and professional expertise, yet poses a higher challenge for the individual practitioner to find his economically viable place among the ever-increasing competition. A positive aspect in the economic environment in which the veterinary profession is operating remains the fact of rising average expenditure per household for all animal species in the past years. For any successful start or reorganization of veterinary entities, it is imperative to closely monitor and consider those developments for future veterinary practice planning.

Moreover, the reasons for failed veterinary practice management due to lack of management and financial knowledge, and skills should be well known in order to avoid those pitfalls and to have good growth and success prospects for a sustainable veterinary business in the future.

REFERENCES

[1]   AVMA (2010a). Reference. Market research statistics. Veterinary specialists – 2006. http://www.avma.org/reference/marketstats/2006/vetspec_2006.asp (Accessed on January 11th, 2011).

[8]   AVMA (2010b). Reference. Market research statistics. Veterinary specialists – 2007. http://www.avma.org/reference/marketstats/2007/vetspec_2007.asp (Accessed on January 11th, 2011).

[9]   AVMA (2010c). Reference. Market research statistics. Veterinary specialists – 2008. http://www.avma.org/reference/marketstats/2008/vetspec_2008.asp (Accessed on January 11th, 2011).

[10] AVMA (2010d). Reference. Market research statistics. Veterinary specialists – 2009. http://www.avma.org/reference/marketstats/vetspec.asp (Accessed on January 11th, 2011).

[11] AVMA (2010e). Reference. U.S. pet ownership – 2001. http://www.avma.org/reference/marketstats/2001/ownership_2001.asp (Accessed on January 11th, 2011).

[12] AVMA (2010f). Reference. U.S. pet ownership – 2007. http://www.avma.org/reference/marketstats/ownership.asp (Accessed on January 11th, 2011).

[13] AVMA (2010g). Reference. Market research statistics. U.S. veterinarians – 2006. http://www.avma.org/reference/marketstats/2006/usvets_2006.asp (Accessed on January 11th, 2011).

[14] AVMA (2010h). Reference. Market research statistics. U.S. veterinarians – 2007. http://www.avma.org/reference/marketstats/2007/usvets_2007.asp (Accessed on January 11th, 2011).

[15] AVMA (2010i). Reference. Market research statistics. U.S. veterinarians – 2008. http://www.avma.org/reference/marketstats/2008/usvets_2008.asp (Accessed on January 11th, 2011).

[16] AVMA (2010j). Reference. Market research statistics. U.S. veterinarians – 2009. http://www.avma.org/reference/marketstats/usvets.asp (Accessed on January 11th, 2011).

[17] Brown, J.P. and Silverman, J.D. (1999). The current and future market for veterinarians and veterinary medical services in the United States. *JAVMA,* Vol. 215, No. 2, July 15. pp. 161-183.

[18] Bureau of Labor Statistics (2010). Occupational outlook handbook, 2010-11 edition. http://www.bls.gov/oco/ocos076.htm . (Accessed on January 11th, 2011).

[19] Chapman, B. (1991). Homoeopathic treatment for birds. *Saffron Walden.* The C.W. Daniel Company Ltd. Essex. UK.

[20] Cron, W.L., Slocum, J.V., Goodnight, D.B. and Volk, J.O. (1999). Impact of management practices and business behaviors on small animal veterinarians; income. *AVMA study.*

[21] Day, Ch. (1998). The homeopathic treatment of small animals. Principles and practice. 4th ed. Saffron Walden. The C.W. Daniel Company Ltd. Essex. UK.

[22] Deutsches Tierärzteblatt (2006). *Einkommenssteuer: Statistik 2001.* 5/2006, pp. 562-564.

[23] Deutsches Tierärzteblatt (2009). *Einkommenssteuer: Statistik2004.* 8/2009, pp. 1036-1037.

[24] Draehmpaehl, D. and Zohmann, A. (1998). Akupunktur bei Hund und Katze. Wissenschaftliche Grundlagen und Praxis. *Ferdinand Enke Verlag, Stuttgart.* Germany.

[25] Dorenkamp, B. (1998). *Natural health care for your bird. Barron's Educational SeriesInc.* New York.

[26] Friedrich, B. and Schäffer, J. (2008). Zur beruflichen und privaten Situation tierärztlicher Praxisassistenten/-innen. *Deutsche Tierärzteblatt.* 1/2008. pp. 4-13.

[27] Megginson, W.L., Byrd, M.J. and Megginson, L.C. (2000). *Small business management: An entrepreneur's guidebook.* 3rd ed. McGraw-Hill. Boston, Madrid, Toronto.

[28] Müller, M.G. and Abu Aabed, A. (2007). Guidelines for setting up a small and medium size enterprise. MBA Thesis, University of Strathclyde. Graduate School of Business. Glasgow, UK.

[29] Ouwerkerk, M. and Schlegel, H. (1997). Erfolgreich Praxisführung für den Tierarzt: Praxismanagament/ Praxismarketing. Hannover. Schlütersche GmbH.

[30] Robertson-Smith, G., Robinson, D., Hicks, B., Khambhaita, P. and Hayday, S. (2010). The 2010 RCVS survey of the UK veterinary and veterinary nursing professions. Royal College of Veterinary Surgeons (RCVS), November 2010. http://www.employment-studies.co.uk/pubs/report.php?id=rcvs1110. (Accessed on January 11th, 2011).

[31] Robinson, D. and Hooker, H. (2006). The UK veterinary profession in 2006. The findings of a survey of the profession conducted by the Royal College of Veterinary Surgeons.

[32] Shilcock, M. and Stutchfield, G. (2005). Veterinary practice management. *A practical guide.* Reprinted, Saunders, Elsevier Ltd. Philadelphia.

[33] Sonnenschmidt, R. and Wagner, M. (1996). Vögel. Akupunktur. Homöopathie. Bachblütentherapie. Kinesiologie. Verlag Eugen Ulmer GmbH&Co. Stuttgart. Germany.

[34] Vetline (2006). Lernen von den Besten. June 31st. http://www.vetline.de/vetservices/ praxismanager/geld_und_recht/benchmarking.htm (Accessed on October 11th, 2006).

[35] Walter, R. (2003). Why business education is important. Veterinary Practice. http://www.vmba.biz.you/bized.htm (Accessed on October 11th, 2006).

[36] Ziffus, G. (2001). Existenzgründung Tierarztpraxis. *Parey Buchverlag.* Berlin. Germany.

[37] Ziffus, G. and Dolle, S. (2000). Marketing und Management in der tierärztlichen Praxis. *Parey Buchverlag.* Berlin. Germany.

Chapter 3

MARKET ANALYSIS

ABSTRACT

A thorough and complete market analysis is a fundamental part of the setting up of a brand new veterinary practice or buying a new practice. The analysis should comprise the premises, location, environment and infrastructure as well as any potential customer groups. Within the market analysis, the customer analysis plays a very important as it enables the prospective veterinary entity owner to gain a better understanding of the potential customer clientele of the veterinary practice. Equally important is the compilation of a thorough and detailed competitor analysis as a major component for a successful and professional practice planning and management.

3.1. INTRODUCTION

In order to prepare a business plan for setting up a new veterinary practice or to purchase an established practice, it is highly essential to conduct a thorough market analysis. This requires detailed definitions and information on the market itself, its definition in the particular case, thorough market research and potential market segmentation. The customer analysis should comprise customer profiling and the definition of potential customer groups as well as an analysis of the customer base. As any business operates in a competitive environment, any market analysis would not be complete without a meticulous competitor analysis. Then individual points are detailed below.

3.2. MARKET DEFINITION AND MARKET RESEARCH

3.2.1. Market Definition

The market is defined as a place where consumers and sellers meet in a specially defined market location [1] or meeting place [6]. Another definition for market is "a place where a product might be sold" as well as "the groups of people who might buy a product" [4, p.124].

For veterinary entities this means the catchment area of the customer target group which could be a town, suburb, a range of housing blocks or a radius of X miles depending on the spread of potential customers and their animals.

3.2.2. Market Research

It is well-known that "research is the cornerstone of any successful business venture" [12, p.40]. This is very much true as many mistakes and business failures could be easily avoided by conducting extensive research before the setting up [7]. Market research needs to be done in a structured approach [12] not only for the multinational business world, but for any small businesses set up as well [7].

Usually, market research is divided into primary and secondary research. Primary research comprises two types of research: explanatory and specific research. Explanatory research has an open-ended structure whereas specific research has a very well defined scope and is of a problem- solving nature. Usually primary research is conducted through questionnaires or interviews whereas secondary research includes study of published data, statistics, journals, etc. [12]. In the small enterprise field, primary research can be done by questioning consumers, potential competitors and business clients. Especially helpful for business research and therefore, also for veterinary practices are population statistics, registration lists of the inhabitants of a city, specialized business magazines and journals. Information about changes in the business market can be gathered from the professional associations [7], newspaper articles and advertisement of services of competitors as well as the observation of trends in human medicine and associated fields.

3.2.3. Market Segmentation

Market segmentation is "the identification of individuals or organizations with similar characteristics that have significant implications for the determination of marketing strategy" [5, p.210]. The market is split in related smaller sub-markets in order to understand and serve the customer in a more efficient way by adding sub-market specific extra services. Those smaller markets cater to the special requirements of customers, while at the same time increasing the profit of the business. The advantages of undertaking market segmentation are manifold, ranging from the selection of the target market, establishing of differential marketing strategies, setting up a tailor-made marketing, product and services mix to evaluating the opportunities and threats to the small enterprise [5].

3.3. CUSTOMER ANALYSIS

The customer analysis can gather data about the customer himself/herself and his or her requirements [12]. Moreover, it helps greatly to understand the customer when developing customer scenarios as business models. This approach can even help to get innovate ideas for the business. One of the major issues is to identify a target customer as well as his or her particular situation in dealing with the company [10].

3.3.1. Customer Groups and Profile

The customer profiling is highly important for the success of not only small businesses and can be achieved through consumer marketing segmentation [5]. Information about the customer type, product or service type, purchasing power, demographic situation, required services/products, additional services/products, customer behavior is essential [9] as the more information can be gathered about the practice customer clientele, the more tailor-made services can be offered to the customers.

Customers can be divided in three groups, the primary target customer, the secondary target customer and the invisible target customer. The primary target customer can be regarded as a heavy user or repeated customer [9]. In terms of veterinary entities, this would be the animal owner who would loyally have treated the patient throughout its lifetime by one particular veterinarian or veterinary entity thus building a personal relationship with the veterinary staff. By contrast, some clients are defined as the secondary target customer being not a frequent one. This is the group of animal owners who frequently change their veterinarians due to actual or imagined complaints or the advice of fellow animal owners. An often unrealized customer group is the so-called invisible target customer. This is the client who is not visible to the opening of the business but may appear later, posing a new market opportunity [9]. It may be that this potential clientele does not have an animal at the time of opening and may be induced to 'try' the vet by word of mouth after acquiring one.

3.3.2. Customer Base Analysis

For the veterinary market, the customer base might include persons who want to buy a pet for the first time and seek advice from the veterinarian before the purchase. Moreover, it can include a pet owner who asks for grooming services or nutritional advice.

When looking at the veterinarians and population relation, e.g. in Germany, one practicing veterinarian has a market share of 10,000 persons. In Switzerland, it is solely 7,000 and in Austria only 6,000 persons [8]. This is not a high number as this number includes non-pet owners and pet owners alike. In the U.S., an area population of 4,000 was suggested as adequate customer base for one veterinarian [3]. Other sources suggest that 70,000 persons living in one residence area are highly sufficient for one veterinary clinic [13]. A radius of 15 minutes travel time by car can be regarded as the catchment area for a newly established veterinary practice [3].

The age factor of pet owners should not be underestimated as the 65+ generation is on the rise as important customer base. Statistical research mentions an increase of market share for veterinary services from 11.5% in 1990 to 51.4% in 2000 for the 65+ household. For pet services like boarding or grooming the number of 65+ customers rose from 10.4% in 1990 to 58% in 2000 [3].

However, customers choose their veterinarian according to his character, information provided, high-quality care reputation, past experiences, variety of services, location and opening hours as well as a recommendation [2].

3.4. COMPETITOR ANALYSIS

3.4.1. Competitor Worksheet

A small and medium-size business has competitors like any other business entity, and they need to be carefully evaluated in order to estimate possible negative influences on the new business set up. For this purpose, a useful tool in profiling and understanding the respective competitors is a competitor worksheet [9].

This should comprise all important data like:

- Personal data - competitor's name, business name, address;
- Business data - length of business existence, market share, target customer profiles, consumer profiles, image and reputation, and if available official financial data in case of public or semi public large clinic groups;
- Service data - the range of offered services, pricing structure, marketing, special customer services, strengths, weaknesses.

From the competitor worksheet information, a 'competitor matrix' can be established. The competitor matrix compares all competitors in one chart, which will help in identifying the ranking and importance of the competitors. When looking at the competitor worksheet, different kinds of competitors can be identified. They can be divided into three main groups [12]:

- Direct competitors with similar setup and skills
- Secondary competitors with some common setup and skills
- Indirect competitors with no direct influence on competition

The competitors for veterinary practices have to be analyzed in the same way as it is applicable to a small and medium-size enterprise. Competitor worksheets can be tailor-made for the special requirements and situation of the veterinary practice. The table below may serve as an example for such a tailor-made competitor worksheet for veterinary practices.

Direct competitors are all veterinary practices with the same specialization, e.g. small animals in the respective area. This can lead to a considerable pressure, especially in very popular areas like big cities. Secondary competitors are e.g. pet shops, which sell pet food, pet accessories, pet vitamins and pet medicines as well as live pets. In the past years, a large number of pet hypermarkets have emerged as strong competition like the franchise Fressnapf in Germany. Those pet hypermarkets allow pets to enter the market, and all pet accessories for sale can be tried on the pets. Pets can even try different food brands in order to give the owners the right choice of food to buy. Many veterinary practices have a small pet shop integrated with a limited range of the most important pet foods which often does not have competitive prices due to the limited number of sales and range of items [7].

The internet can be regarded as indirect competitors for veterinary practices. More and more, veterinarians offer their services via the internet as internet consultation or veterinary online advice [7]. Moreover, an increasing number of pet medicines and vitamins are sold on the internet nowadays [11] because this distribution way saves the consultation fees, and it sells items cheaper. Equally important, the internet sale of veterinary products has reached global dimensions and has opened new markets [7].

Table 3.1. Sample competitor worksheet for the veterinary practice

	Competitor A (direct competitor)	Competitor B (secondary competitor)	Competitor C (indirect competitor)
Where is the practice of your competitors located?			
Since when are your competitors in business?			
What is the competitors' market share?			
What are the target customers?			
What are the annual sales of the competitors?			
How is the competitors' reputation?			
What are their main services?			
What is their price structure?			
What is their marketing?			
What are their strengths?			
What are their weaknesses?			
Is their practice expanding?			
Is their practice loosing market shares?			
What are their special customer services?			

3.5. PORTER'S FIVE FORCES MODEL

Another useful model to understand the competitors and the competitive business structure is the Porter's 'Five Forces' model. One of those five forces is the entry barriers towards other competitors thus reducing their chances to enter the market. Another force is the bargaining power of the suppliers which may be a major issue for small businesses. However, the bargaining power of the buyers is also not a major factor contributing to competition as the quantity of products bought is not so high in small businesses. The fourth force, the threat of substitutes, does affect the small and medium-size business to a great extent if highly specialized niche products and services are provided uniquely by the small businesses. The last major force is the intensity of rivalry between competitors, which might affect the small businesses if they are in a field where a larger number of businesses exists [5].

One advantage of the Porter's Five Forces model is the fact that it helps to understand the value-sharing and profit redistribution. It widens the look at competitors as it goes beyond the direct competitors for a veterinary practice which means other veterinary practices. Another advantage is that this model also gives ideas about a wider context, including the external practice environment than just to evaluate the service range of the veterinary practice.

3.6. CONCLUSION

Veterinarians need to obtain a working knowledge about business tools like market analysis and competitor studies and not shy away from utilizing them to the advantage of their business. This may help significantly to avoid major pitfalls and become a key to successful veterinary practice establishment and management. It has been a proven helpful strategy to revisit these analyses from time to time like annually or bi-annually after setting up or buying the veterinary practice as market conditions and competitors might change. If changing markets, customer base and competitor groups are not taken into consideration, a major negative impact on the veterinary practice business may arise. A late reaction thereof could be too late to correct the situation in a positive way. It is by far easier to adjust one's strategy to any changed situation right from the beginning than being forced to react after new competitors have established themselves in one's home market and taken over part of one's customers.

REFERENCES

[1]   Bannock, G., Davis, I., Trott, P. and Uncles, M. (2002). The new penguin dictionary of business. *Penguin books.* London. England.

[2]   Brown, J.P. and Silverman, J.D. (1999). The current and future market for veterinarians and veterinary medical services in the United States. *JAVMA*, Vol. 215, No. 2, July 15. pp. 161-183.

[3]   Catanzaro, T.E. (1998). Building the successful veterinary practice: programs and procedures. Wiley-Blackwell.

[4]   Collin, P.H. (2003). Dictionary of economics. *Bloomsdury Publishing.* London. England.

[5]   Jobber, D. (2004). Principles and practice of marketing. 4th ed. McGraw-Hill Int. Ltd. Berkshire, UK.

[6]   Lines, D., Marcouse, I. and Martin, P. (1999). The complete A-Z business studies handbook. 2nd ed. *Hodder and Stoughton.* Tottenham. London.

[7]   Müller, M.G. and Abu Aabed, A. (2007). Guidelines for setting up a small and medium size enterprise. MBA Thesis, University of Strathclyde. Graduate School of Business. Glasgow, UK.

[8]   Ouwerkerk, M. and Schlegel, H. (1997). Erfolgreich Praxisführung für den Tierarzt: Praxismanagament/ Praxismarketing. Hannover. Schlütersche GmbH.

[9]   Ryan, J.D. and Hiduke, G.P. (2006). Small business: an entrepreneur's business plan. 7th ed. Thompson South-Western. Ohio.

[10]   Seybold, P.B. (2001). Get inside the lives of your customers. Harvard Business Review, May. pp.81-89.

[11]   Shilcock, M. and Stutchfield, G. (2005). Veterinary practice management. *A practical guide*. Reprinted, Saunders, Elsevier Ltd. Philadelphia.

[12]   The Entrepreneur Magazine (1999). Small business advisor. 2nd ed. John Entrepreneur Media Inc. Wiley&Sons. New York, Chichester, Weinheim, Brisbane, Singapore, Toronto.

[13]   Vetline (2006). Quo vadis, Tierarztpraxis? July 9th. http://www.vetline.de/vetservices/ praxismanager/geld_und_recht/standortanalyse_tierarztpraxis.htm   (Accessed   on October 11th, 2006).

Chapter 4

VETERINARY PRACTICE TYPES

ABSTRACT

As veterinary entities are businesses, they may be founded under different legal statuses. The type of veterinary practice types may range from single ownership practices, partnership practices or even franchised veterinary practices under a limited liability company status in some countries. All veterinary business types can be compared to small and medium-sized enterprises. For this reason, this chapter focuses on the different types of small and medium enterprises in general and then applies their characteristics to the various veterinary practice types. This breakdown is important as it enhances the understanding of a veterinary practice as a business and not just as a veterinary medical establishment. Often, the business idea gets lost in the context of specific veterinary issues, making it more difficult for veterinarians to immerse themselves deeper in the business world.

4.1. INTRODUCTION

When talking about setting up a veterinary practice, usually the entity will start as a small business requiring the same management tools as larger or more mature entities [14, 17]. Between 64% and 85% of the veterinarians are working in private practices [4, 17] thus making it to the most favorite working environment for veterinarians. Out of those, 10-15% are practice associates in European countries like Germany, Switzerland and Austria [17]. This has manifold implications not only on the veterinary market, but also on the business side of veterinary practices.

4.2. DEFINITIONS OF SME (SMALL AND MEDIUM SIZE ENTERPRISE)

The choice of the right business and the right start into the entrepreneurial work life is one of the major factors for success. The US Congress in the Small Business Act of 1953 has defined "a small business is one that is independently owned and operated and is not dominant in its field of operation" [14, p.11].

Very small businesses are defined as companies with fewer than 20 employees [14]. Small businesses are regarded as businesses with less than 100 employees [25, 32]. They form about 20 million businesses in the USA with one million new small business start-up's yearly and 7 million potential future entrepreneurs [25]. Medium-size businesses meanwhile are companies with 100 to 499 employees [14].

According to research [14], small businesses also have to fall under at least two out of four qualitative factors as:

- Independent management with the manager being usually the owner of the company
- Supplied capital, ownership of one or few persons
- Local operation area (market does not have to be local)
- Small business compared to other competing companies in the industry sector

4.3. ROLE OF SMES IN THE ECONOMY

According to former U.S. President Ronald Reagan, "The good health and strength of America's small businesses are a vital key to the health and strength of our economy… Indeed, small business is America." [14, p.2]. In the USA, SMEs can be regarded as one of the major driving forces behind the growth and vitality of the U.S. economy. According to the U.S. Bureau of the Census, small businesses represent over 97 percent of all businesses in the United States, having an annual payroll above $1 trillion [32]. SMEs have found their way in all different parts of the economy and are a vital driver of integrating persons of various social, racial, ethnic, religious and sexual backgrounds [32], and they offer excellent opportunities, especially for women and older workers [14]. In the USA, every third household is involved in a small business, and in the private sector, the majority of new jobs are set up in companies with less than 20 employees [25]. It is estimated that in 1996 64% out of 2.5 million new jobs in the U.S. were created in SMEs [14]. This shows the tremendous economic importance of SMEs in the modern business world.

Small and medium-size enterprises offer some special advantages to their employees such as greater job motivation and job satisfaction as well as a comprehensive learning experience. The reason is that employees have to perform more tasks and jobs than in larger, highly specialized companies. Moreover, small businesses have a greater innovation and flexibility and direct close relationship to their customers [14].

4.4. BUSINESS MODELS F SMES

Small and medium-size enterprises can be small shops of one family, but also multiple unit businesses [32]. Different business models of SMEs exist ranging from sole ownership businesses, joint partnership businesses to franchise.

4.4.1. Single Business Ownership

Single ownerships pose a wide range of advantages and disadvantages, which are explained in more detail in table 4.1. The big advantages are the decision-making power and keeping of the profit, as well as the direct contact with the market. However, the limited financial resources pose major problems as do the long working hours and sole risk taking inherent in sole ownership. Other problems can include the self-responsible decision-making and deficiencies in managerial skills [6, 31].

Table 4.1. Advantages and Disadvantages of Sole Business Ownership [modified from 6, 31]

Sole Business Ownership	
Advantages	Disadvantages
Own decision-making => can lead to higher motivation	Limited sources of finance
Quickly decision-making => rapid response to changes in the market	Relies heavily on his or her own ability to make decisions
Direct contact with the market	Long working hours, limited holidays => increased stress level
Easy setting up	Unlimited liability
Keeps all the rewards	Often limited managerial skills
Privacy of business affairs	No one to share ideas with

4.4.2. Joint Ownership Business

In a joint ownership business, the risk is equally distributed to more than one person. More financial resources can be made available and ideas, and knowledge can be shared better, and the respective partners can share their work load and can cover each other during leave or further specialization.

Table 4.2. Advantages and Disadvantages of Joint Ownership Business [modified from 6, 31]

Joint Partnership Business	
Advantages	Disadvantages
Limited liability	Payment of the registering costs
Can raise finance from selling shares	Has to make the accounts public
Is often perceived as being more established than sole owners	Payment for the yearly accounts audit
Share resources / ideas / knowledge	Has to disclose information
Can cover for each other, e.g. during holidays	Subject to company law i.e. greater regulation than a sole trader
More sources of finance than sole owner	Shared profits between partners
Partners can specialize better	Slower decision making than sole owner

However, at the same time, the decision-making process and profits have to be shared, and information has to be disclosed. More legal requirements and restraints might lead to further disadvantages in the joint ownership business [6, 31]. Further advantages and disadvantages can be seen in Table 4.2.

4.4.3. Franchising

4.4.3.1. Definition and History

Franchising is defined as a relationship on a continuous basis between franchisor (franchisor company) and franchisee with the responsibility of the provision to do business and support in organizing, training and management by a licensed way [12]. The franchisor gives the license to use his brand name and to sell his services or products to the franchisee being an independent business owner who has to pay fees and royalties [24, 36]. Franchises can be divided into four groups - manufacturing franchises, product franchises, business format franchises and business opportunities franchise [12]. Today mobile specialty franchising especially in the services' sector, is on the rise [20].

Moreover, franchising covers a wide range of national and international business systems through contractual franchise agreements. Legal obligations exist for both parties like liability of franchisors for their franchisees [15]. However, in international franchising, cultural distances and differences should not be underestimated. This might lead to a re-arrangement of the franchise set up [2] like the adoption of "flexible organizational arrangements that permit the use of country-specific knowledge" [26, p.500]. At the same time, not all geographic areas provide the same chances for franchisors [7].

Early forms of franchising date back to the Middle Age when the tax collector collected money on behalf of the Catholic Church and kept a percentage of it [21]. However, in modern times the first franchising operation in the early 1850s was Singer Company, which sold sewing machines [36]. This franchising approach failed, but did not prevent other companies from successfully following this path, such as the Coca-Cola company established by John S. Pemberton in 1886 [21]. In 1902, David Liggett paved the way for modern franchising by setting up a drug cooperative of several pharmacists under the name "Rexall", the first franchising chain. The real rise of franchising came after the second world war and today every 12th business in the USA is a franchising operation with a volume of $1 trillion in the 1990s [21].

4.4.3.2. Advantages and Disadvantages

Franchising provides certain advantages for the franchisor like rapid business expansion, increased profits and enhanced distribution networks with little financial investment [36] as well as an established operation method and marketing campaigns [21]. Satisfied franchisees will be the key asset for successful franchising operations resulting in high profits [30].

The franchise model provides the chance for a good business start with a reputed brand name and business support provided by the franchisor [36], reducing startup risk and improving the chances of securing bank loans [21]. Moreover, franchising offers a good growth strategy for small businesses [10]. Customers benefit from the franchising chains by getting exactly the same proven services or products anywhere [36].

One disadvantage of franchising is that the franchisors can suffer from incompetent franchisees [36]. Other problems may arise when a franchisor is growing too fast without a good business foundation [29]. On the other side, franchisees cannot develop their own identity [21] and are not in control of their business as they must fit in the franchisor's operational business system [36], and must closely follow the guidelines and orders of the franchisor [21].

4.4.3.3. Veterinary Franchising

The first veterinary franchise company was established in 1955 by Banfield, the Pet Hospital®. However, the breakthrough came only after teaming up with PetSmart® being the largest pet shop in the USA through opening in-store veterinary clinics [3]. In 2003, Banfield started the international franchising of veterinary hospitals in the UK, followed by another expansion to Mexico in 2005 [3] by selling franchise licenses between US $242,000 and US $443,000 per franchise operation [9].

Nowadays, Medical Management International operating under the Banfield brand name has emerged as the largest veterinary hospital franchisor worldwide with more than 670 national and international franchised locations, yearly revenue of 187,5 million US$ [37] and 7,000 employees among them 2,250 veterinarians [8].

Apart from other competitors which sell pet medicines and products over the internet like PetMed Express [19], Drs. Foster & Smith [5], PetCareRx.com [18] and KV Vet Supply Company [11], the main competitor for Banfield in the veterinary franchise market is VCA Antech.

VCA Antech provides pet health care systems to its network of 540 veterinary hospitals as well as laboratory services to its own hospital and 14,000 small animal hospitals in the USA with its own clinical laboratory, Antech Diagnostics [34].

More franchise companies try to put their foot into this lucrative doorstep like Echo Healthcare, which has bought XLNT Veterinary Care with the aim to "become a dominant national provider of veterinary primary health care services" [1].

4.5. ISSUES RELATED TO STARTING A SME

People start a new business because they believe that they have found a good business opportunity. However, their business idea has to be tested against the main questions of having a competitive advantage over their competitors, and the idea will only work as business if there is demand for the product or service, and the idea is profitable. In addition, the new entrepreneur needs to assess the required skills and abilities for the realization of the business idea [31].

The most important issue at the start of a small business is analysis, analysis and again analysis of both, yourself and your environment. Furthermore, it is highly important to set the right and achievable objectives and goals [32] for the business right from the start of the planning phase. This applies in the same way to every veterinary practice or hospital.

4.5.1. Assessment

The personal analysis should include the personal potential, abilities and skills [14] as well as the professional and financial knowledge and ability as detailed below [13].

4.5.1.1. Personal Assessment

The personal assessment should also cover the personal motivation for setting up a business [13]. This includes the right motivation for setting up a business; it is not sufficient motivation just to be frustrated with the current job to decide to start ones' own practice. Strong motivation is required on a long-term basis because a lot of obstacles will have to be faced, especially the first two years after the opening of a new enterprise which can be quite demanding and difficult in terms of acquiring a loyal clientele and financial-wise. The personal strengths and weaknesses have to be thoroughly evaluated.

A business owner depends largely on himself in the daily routine and is the most important focal point for the customer. Therefore, he needs to have a pleasant personality with good communication skills in order to establish a strong relationship with his client. Moreover, a potential business owner needs to be prepared to work extended hours and weekends, as well as refraining from long holidays, which can have a high impact on his social and family life. Therefore, the support of the family must be ensured as this is one of the critical success factors for a small business. Good organizing skills, stamina and strong health are other contributing factors for success [16].

4.5.1.2. Professional Assessment

Professional skills, abilities and motivation need to be clearly assessed. This includes not only the professional experience, but also characteristics like team work, perseverance and good decision-making skills. Equally important are well developed listening and negotiation skills, managerial ability and the establishment of priorities. Moreover, developing a vision of the future business along with objectives, goals and business strategy are essential in the professional assessment [35]. Financial and managerial planning skills will greatly help in establishing and managing a successful veterinary practice. Fundamentally, any business idea can only work out if there is sufficient demand for the products or services [31].

The professional assessment covers good experience in diagnosis and treatment of pets. Pet owners can very well evaluate the experience of the veterinarian as this shows clearly in the way how he deals with their pet. Only when they are convinced about the abilities and knowledge of the veterinarian, they will build up trust and confidence being prerequisites for a loyal customer clientele. A major asset for a newly opened veterinary practice might be a specialization by species (e.g. felines, birds, reptiles, small rodents) or subject (e.g. dentistry, dermatology, surgery) which are new emerging features in the current market situation [28]. Team work ability as well as leadership qualities are essential as there is usually different staff (e.g. receptionist, veterinary technicians, assistant) working in a veterinary practice with different education background, character and experiences. Management abilities and knowledge are one of the most important factors for success but mostly not available at the time of setting up the practice. During the veterinary studies at university, management and business are not taught as part of the curriculum. Later while working as assistant in a veterinary practice, the veterinarian does not have much contact with these subjects as mostly the practice owner will deal with these issues [16].

4.5.1.3. Financial Assessment

The financial assessment should include the financial resources such as the existing capital [13]. Personal capital can include cash money, savings, bonds, funds or shares. Another way of securing capital is loans from family members or friends. However, care needs to be taken on the legal side, and clear contracts are required. In order to overcome the low-income opening phase of the business, it might be extremely helpful to have a second income in the family, e.g. by the spouse, as this can remove the day-to-day pressure of family financial maintenance needs [16].

Table 4.3. Assessment requirements for potential business owners [16]

Personal assessment	Professional assessment	Financial assessment
● Motivations for setting up a business	● Good and extensive professional experience	● Personal capital
● Strengths and weaknesses	● Possible specialization or niche	● Bonds, funds, shares
● Preparedness to work long hours and at weekends	● Relationship with customers	● Loan from family members or friends
● Preparedness to refrain from long holidays	● Team work ability	● Second income in the family
● Support of the family	● Leadership qualities	● Monthly required income
● Communication skills	● Management abilities and knowledge	
● Organizing skills		

4.5.1.4. Quality Certifications

The next step after the analysis is the planning phase. A good planning can save your business and make it successful. However, for veterinary practices quality certifications, planning or control is not yet mandatory like ISO certifications for manufacturing companies. In the UK, an approach called "Good Veterinary Practice" has started to establish the best practices and good-quality management in veterinary practices although no clear fully accepted unified definition exists until now [33]. Nevertheless, official regulations might come in the future, and in any way quality planning and control help to improve the quality of services in a veterinary practice [16].

4.6. NEW SETTING UP OR BUYING AN ESTABLISHED BUSINESS

4.6.1. Veterinary Practice Structures

After deciding which type of veterinary practice to open, the next important decision is whether to start a new practice or to buy an existing one. Care should be taken, however, when buying an existing business as the reason for the sale needs to be thoroughly evaluated. In UK, the majority of veterinary practices are managed through partnerships 23]. Over the past years, the single veterinarian practice has lost its leading position in the veterinary practice. The current trend in Europe goes to either single ownership with several assistant veterinarians or joint ownerships [17], which has the same major advantages and disadvantages as mentioned before for SMEs in tables 4.1. and 4.2. In the future, a further increase of veterinary practices owned by limited companies or corporate is predicted whereas sole ownership or partnerships as veterinary practice types will further decrease [22].

Table 4.4. Data of practice ownership in UK [23]

Practice Ownership	%
Partnership	50
Sole principal	29
Limited company	15
Charity	3
Corporate concern	2
Other ownerships	2

The numbers of veterinary surgeons are increasing according to a study of Fort Dodge in March 2007 [28].

The practices' types are also changing. The 2006 RCVS survey shows that 25% of veterinary surgeons are working in mixed practice, 45% in small animal/exotic practice and 6% in equine practice. Only 4% of veterinary surgeons work in farm practices and 3% in other practices. However, 6% work in referral practices or consulting [23]. Especially large practices have their clinics located in different sites to cover a larger area.

Table 4.5. Number of veterinary surgeons in veterinary practices [28]

Number of veterinary surgeons	%
< 2	19
2 – 2.9	18
3 – 3.9	20
4 – 4.9	16
5 – 5.9	10
6 – 6.9	6
7 – 7.9	6
8 and above	6

Veterinary practices or hospitals set ups are changing, too. In the UK, in 2005 only 47% of the practices were a single-site practice, but 26% of practices had two sites and another 26% of practices had 3 and more sites [27]. In 2008, the largest group practice in the UK possesses over 100 sites. An average of 40 sites is nowadays normal for corporate or larger group practices [28].

In the USA, the largest privately owned veterinary group owns 670 veterinary clinics [37]. Moreover, corporate veterinary practices are on the jump to the stock market [28]. This development will lead to considerable changes soon in the veterinary practice landscape.

However, it should not be underestimated that it requires sometimes even up to six or seven years to establish a veterinary practice completely in the market [38].

4.6.2. Setting up of a New Veterinary Business

To open a new business right from the scratch requires a lot of efforts, but should be rewarding in the end as it gives the business owner the chance to design the business entirely to his own wishes in the best possible way depending on his budget availability. Another advantage is the free choice of the location of the business as well of the equipment and machinery. Moreover, after finding a suitable location, the premises can be arranged according to the individual business needs [16].

On the other hand, one of the major disadvantages is that the customer clientele needs to be established from zero. This requires a lot of effort, time and marketing. The new business needs to build its reputation and convince the consumers that they will provide the best service for them, which can take years [16].

4.6.3. Buying an Established Business

There are several advantages in the option of buying an existing business. One is that the business has already been successfully established and has a proven record with loyal customer clientele. The equipment is already available and may need only some additional purchases. Often bank loans are easier to get [32] because an existing business will offer a higher security for the bank over a newly established one.

However, there are also disadvantages involved in the purchase of an existing enterprise. One disadvantage can be old and outdated material and equipment; another one might be a poor reputation of the previous owner, or an unsuitable location of the business. The competitor situation needs to be researched carefully as some enterprises are sold when a lot of new competitor firms enter the market.

Sometimes, the seller of the business entity will set up a new one in a close neighborhood, although this can be prevented by a clear contractual agreement [13]. Other problems include the selling price of the business and requirements for taking over staff from the previous enterprise which can lead to difficulties as they are not used to a different way of working [32].

4.6.4. New Veterinary Practice Forms

When setting up a veterinary practice, the direction of the appropriate practice type has to be clear right from the start. A main decision has to be taken whether a purely veterinary practice or a practice with additional services like laboratory, grooming and pet shop will be established [16].

New forms of veterinary practices are referral practices and emergency service clinics. Referral practices perform only referral work and are often highly specialized in e.g. orthopedics or neurology. They have a much wider radius of customer base and liaise very closely with several veterinary practices that are referring their clients to them. In many of those referral practices, university professors and veterinary specialists work either full-time or part-time. This enhances also the general health care system for animals as such a specialist treatment with latest equipment cannot be performed in a general veterinary practice or hospital.

Emergency service clinics have had a major impact on veterinary work life in the past years. Those clinics perform night duties. This is very much to the advantage of general veterinary practices as it reduces their night duties [28]. Although not yet widely distributed in all countries, it has become a new feature in larger cities but does not seem to be a very feasible option in rural areas due to the low number of nightly emergency cases.

For small animal practices, normal routine services include general examinations, dental prevention, and vaccinations. Surgical interventions included neutering and spaying, soft tissue and orthopedic surgery. However, depending on the financial ability and possible specialization, other modules can be added step by step after the practice is well established. Other additional modules might be ultrasound, cardiology or ophthalmology.

The ultrasound can be used for soft-tissue examination as well as cardiologic examination and represents an advanced tool for organ's diseases like liver, kidney or heart problems and pregnancy detection. Moreover, a special dental department will include advanced dental procedures like root canal treatment, corrections of tooth deformation with e.g. brackets, palatinal surgeries and X-Rays [16].

Following research, more than 86% of pet owners prefer a veterinary clinic with integrated pet product shop [16]. The products range from vitamins to pet food like special diet food or food for older pets to pet accessories. The highly preferred products are with 68% vitamins for pets, 64% veterinary medicines, 60% pet food and 52% pet accessories. The veterinary medicines can range from anti flea products to deworming medicines. The pet accessories can include dog collars, shampoo or dog/cat toys. The pet shop is a very good opportunity to make pet owners comfortable and to provide them with the opportunity to purchase those items while waiting for their appointment. This provides an additional source of income and makes clients happy and satisfied as they have to stop only in one shop. The possibility to have the pet shop online as well and to deliver the chosen items via home delivery services is regarded as an attractive option for a stunning 82% of pet owners [16].

Another service for the newly set up veterinary practice can be a boarding facility for cats, dogs and falcons. A "pet-sitting service" is liked by people, especially those who are working or are busy. These additional services can be used by owners who are traveling for vacations or are sick.

The boarding facility will be established in a professional way with separate areas for the different animal species. Moreover, if space allows, it will be good to have a playground area for socializing dogs. In order to help busy owners, a pick-up service for pets can be a competitive advantage compared to other clinics. This business segment can be regarded as an important core practice segment which can give a steady income for the practice. This is especially helpful in the summer months when many people are traveling, and the practice income will be less [16].

Other facilities of the veterinary practice will be a pet grooming, which will provide a regular source of income on a monthly basis. Apart from the grooming part, the groomer will also detect pets' health problems like ear infections or infected wounds, which will require veterinary treatment. Therefore, the veterinary income will be strengthened further [16].

As life is changing, pet owner wishes change, too. 68% of them wish to have wellness and alternative medicine services offered in the veterinary practice thus making it to a strong business segment and core part of a new practice [16]. Wellness for animals includes pediatric/geriatric profiles like special pediatric/geriatric tests and examinations, diet and behavior consultation.

Nutrition consultation can be offered as well as behavioral courses and consultation as behavioral problems are on the rise in pets as previously discussed in the new veterinary trends. This can be extended to dog obedience courses and training. Moreover, massage and physiotherapy especially following surgeries or arthrosis cases are services that can be provided to secure additional income. The alternative medicine segment may feature homeopathy, acupuncture, Reiki as well as Bach's flowers therapy. The big advantage of this veterinary segment is on one hand the increasing popularity among pet owners and on the other hand, the relative low set up and running costs as expensive equipment is not required [16].

When looking at demographics in modern countries, the age pyramid goes to the older generation and will continue to do so in the next decades. This leads to the fact that more elderly people will have pets. Therefore, veterinary practices have to consider that those older pet owners may face difficulties in bringing their pet to the practice themselves. A pick-up and returning service of pets is extremely customer friendly and will increase the customer base among older pet owners. If veterinary surgeons are concerned about the increased costs of transportation, they can establish one day in the week where they have the "pet pick-up day" and collect more pets of older pet owners. This will be perceived as a great customer service and in the same time substantially reduces transportation costs and staff time. Moreover, it can be regarded as an additional new service that can bring increased income to the practice.

4.7. CONCLUSION

Veterinary practices have undergone major changes in the past years. One veterinarian practices have increased to multi veterinarian practices and large chains of franchised veterinary hospitals. Veterinary practices and hospitals have to be regarded as business entities with the respective business-oriented approach. This changing environment has to be taken into consideration when deciding whether to buy an established veterinary practice or setting up a new one.

This decision should be taken under the aspect of small enterprises with the same personal, professional and financial assessments. A well-funded approach to the decision of buying an established veterinary practice or setting up a brand-new one has to be taken. Recent practice forms include e.g. wellness, alternative medicine, integrated pet shops, grooming and boarding facilities. They can provide a considerable source of income for the veterinary practice.

A sustainable decision for a future successful veterinary entity set up can only be taken with proper assessments and profound information about the changing veterinary practice world.

REFERENCES

[1] Adler, N. (2006). Echo Healthcare to buy veterinary hospital operator. *Washington Business Journal.* September 11. http://www.bizjournals.com/bosotn/othercities/ washington/stories/2006/09/11/dailys.html (Accessed on September 25th, 2006).

[2] Altinay, L. (2004). Implementing international franchising: the role of intrapreneurship. *International Journal of Service Industry Management.* Vol. 15, No. 5. pp. 426-443.

[3] Banfield, (2006). Banfield, The Pet Hospital – Treating your pets like family. http://www.banfield.net/about/mission.asp (Accessed on September 25th, 2006).

[4] Brown, J.P. and Silverman, J.D. (1999). The current and future market for veterinarians and veterinary medical services in the United States. *JAVMA*, Vol. 215, No. 2, July 15. pp. 161-183.

[5] Drs. Foster & Smith (2006). Inc. company profile. http://biz.yahoo.ic/100/100347.html (Accessed on September 25th, 2006).

[6] Gillespie, A. (1998). Advanced Business Studies through diagrams. Oxford University Press. UK.

[7] Hoffmann, R.C. and Preble, J.F. (2004). Global franchising: current status and future challenges. *Journal of Services Marketing.* Vol. 18, No. 2. pp. 101-113.

[8] Hoovers (2011). Medical Management International, Inc http://www.hoovers.com/ company/Medical_Management_International_Inc/rrrcrti-1-1njdap.html (Accessed on August 10th, 2011).

[9] Kim, L.B. (2005). Evaluating a franchise before taking the plunge. Startup Journal. http://www.startupjournal.com/franchising/franchising/20050930-spors.html (Accessed on September 29th, 2006).

[10] Kirby, D. and Watson, A. (1999). Franchising as a small business development strategy: a qualitative study of operational and 'failed' franchisors in the UK. *Journal of Small Business Enterprise Development,* Vol. 6, No. 4. pp. 314-349.

[11] KV Vet Supply Company (2006). Company profile. http://biz.yahoo.ic/110/ 110106.html (Accessed on September 25th, 2006).

[12] Ludden, La Verne L. (1999). *Franchise Opportunities Handbook.* Indianapolis, IN: JIST Works, Inc., Maynard, Roberta.

[13] McMullan, D. (2002). Be your own boss. 3rd ed. *The Sunday Times.* Kogan Page Ltd. London.

[14] Megginson, W.L., Byrd, M.J. and Megginson, L.C. (2000). Small business management: *An entrepreneur's guidebook.* 3rd ed. McGraw-Hill. Boston, Madrid, Toronto.

[15] Morgan, F.W. and Stoltman, J.J. (1997). Vicarious franchisor liability: marketing and public policy implications. *Journal of Business & Industrial Marketing,* Vol. 12, No. 5. pp. 297-314.

[16] Müller, M.G. and Abu Aabed, A. (2007). Guidelines for setting up a small and medium size enterprise. MBA Thesis, University of Strathclyde. *Graduate School of Business.* Glasgow, UK.

[17] Ouwerkerk, M. and Schlegel, H. (1997). Erfolgreich Praxisführung für den Tierarzt: Praxismanagament/ Praxismarketing. Hannover. Schlütersche GmbH.

[18] PetCareRx.com (2006). Inc. company profile. http://biz.yahoo.ic/110/110154.html (Accessed on September 25th, 2006).

[19] PetMed Express (2006). Inc. company profile. http://biz.yahoo.ic/108/108843.html (Accessed on September 25th, 2006).

[20] Preble, J.F. and Hoffmann, R.C. (1998). Competitive advantage through specialty franchising. *Journal of Consumer Marketing*. Vol. 15, No. 1. pp. 64-77.

[21] Reference for Business (2006). Encyclopedia of business, 2nd ed. http://www.referenceforbusiness.com/encyclopedia/For-Gol/Franchising.html (Accessed on September 29th, 2006).

[22] Robertson-Smith, G., Robinson, D., Hicks, B., Khambhaita, P. and Hayday, S. (2010). The 2010 RCVS survey of the UK veterinary and veterinary nursing professions. Royal College of Veterinary Surgeons (RCVS), November 2010. http://www.employment-studies.co.uk/pubs/report.php?id=rcvs1110. (Accessed on January 11th, 2011).

[23] Robinson, D. and Hooker, H. (2006). The UK veterinary profession in 2006. The findings of a survey of the profession conducted by the Royal College of Veterinary Surgeons.

[24] Rubin, P. (1978). The theory of the firm and the structure of the franchise contract. *Journal of Law Economics*. Vol. 21, pp. 223-233.

[25] Ryan, J.D. and Hiduke, G.P. (2006). Small business: an entrepreneur's business plan. 7th ed. Thompson South-Western. Ohio.

[26] Sashi, C.M. and Karuppur, D.P. (2002). Franchising in global markets: towards a conceptual framework. *International Marketing Review*. Vol. 19, No. 5. pp. 499-524.

[27] Shilcock, M. and Stutchfield, G. (2005). Veterinary practice management. A practical guide. Reprinted, Saunders, Elsevier Ltd. Philadelphia.

[28] Shilcock, M. and Stutchfield, G. (2008). Veterinary practice management. A practical guide. 2nd ed. Reprinted, Saunders, Elsevier Ltd. Philadelphia.

[29] Spors, K.K. (2006). For franchises, growing rapidly isn't always best. *Startup Journal*. http://www.startupjournal.com/franchising/franchising/20050930-spors.html (Accessed on September 29th, 2006).

[30] Stites, E. (2006). Satisfaction is everything. Franchising World. September. http://www.franchisebusinessreview.com/Advice/Articles/satisfaction-is-everything.aspx (Accessed on September 29th, 2006).

[31] Surridge, M. and Gillespie, A. (2005). AS Business Studies. Hodder & Stoughton.

[32] The Entrepreneur Magazine (1999). Small business advisor. 2nd ed. John Entrepreneur Media Inc. Wiley&Sons. New York, Chichester, Weinheim, Brisbane, Singapore, Toronto.

[33] The Veterinary Record (2006). *What constitutes good practice?* Vol. 158. no. 2. January 14th, 2006. p. 37.

[34] VCA Antech (2011). VCA Antech. http://www.vcaantech.com.htm (Accessed on August 20th, 2011).

[35] Walker, J. (2006). Managing and leading people. Workshop. Ross University of Michigan Business School. Dubai, 6-8. November.

[36] Wikipedia (2006). Franchising. http://en.wikipedia.org/wiki/Franchising (Accessed on September 29th, 2006).

[37] Wikipedia (2011). Banfield. http://en.wikipedia.org/wiki/Banfield_(pet_hospitals) (Accessed on August 10th, 2011).

[38] Ziffus, G. (2001). Existenzgründung Tierarztpraxis. Parey Buchverlag. Berlin. Germany.

Chapter 5

PLANNING AND STRATEGY

ABSTRACT

Methodical business planning and strategy seems alien to the vast majority of veterinary practice owners or practice managers as only recently modern management tools and practices have found their entry in veterinary practices. The job profile of a "veterinary practice manager" is a very new position that was formerly be held by the practice owner. Although special training for the veterinary practice managers has emerged in several countries like the US and UK, issues had been created due to lacking knowledge of veterinary practice processes and structures. Very rarely do veterinarians hold Master of Business Administration that would provide them with in-depth knowledge of how to run a veterinary practice successfully as a modern small business enterprise. A important tool of modern business practices is a well-planned business plan in connection with a short- and medium-term forecast as well as a clear strategy to provide the veterinary practice with a future-oriented path and clear set objectives. At least basic planning tools should be implemented in every veterinary practice to compare the actual situation with the original goals set. In this chapter, the business strategy and business planning process will be explained in a step-by-step approach. Moreover, a sample business plan is available in this chapter.

5.1. INTRODUCTION

In many professions like in medical professions, theories are an inevitable part of professional work. Without proper theoretical background, no practical work can be performed in the daily real life. This applies also to the setting up of the veterinary business. But how is it for veterinary practitioners where a formal business education is often missing and even for MBAs the difference in their theoretical background is immense? Is it enough just to have the desire to open a new veterinary practice?

Do we really need theories in management in order to become better managers or do we have to rely solely on our intuition and gut feeling? [6]. The best way of tackling this issue is a step-by-step approach and understanding the individual parts of the business planning process. The essential part of business planning is to ask the following questions:

- What do I want to do?
- Where do I want to do it?
- How do I want to do it?
- With whom do I want to do it?
- How much will it cost?
- How can I finance it?

This process includes an easy way to establish a matching strategy for setting up the veterinary practice. First of all, the clear business idea has to be established. Then the necessary start-up costs have to be calculated, and staff requirements identified. This leads to the formal part of setting up a veterinary business: making the well-structured business plan.

This helps not only in getting possible investors or banks on board to fund a new or existing veterinary practice but also aids the veterinary practice owner and his practice manager in reviewing current business processes and comparing them with forecasts. Business plans should not be regarded as static plans as they have to be adjusted to match and reflect current business changes. However, they are an excellent tool to look really at the business from all different perspectives and to get a complete picture.

5.2. THEORY AND PRACTICE – TWO WORLDS APART

The relationship of theory and practice has been regarded as marriage where "theory and practice are two halves of a whole" [4, p.10] showing a strong interaction between both. However, do theories really cope with the daily life requirements of veterinary practices? From our experience, in many cases in reality, they do not [6]. Theories are often unsuitable and cannot be transformed into real-life benefits. Moreover, they are just a large number of words with which they try to explain the world, but fail to give good guidance for inexperienced managers. Moreover, theories do not have to be right or beneficial for a business. Veterinary practitioners and practice managers need to learn to critically assess and differentiate which theories might be helpful for improving their particular situation and, which are entirely useless, waste of time and might even be counterproductive for the business by directly reducing their competitive advantage. It does not help to run blindly behind some prominent and popular theories because each business has different requirements, which need to be seen as priority. However, often managers do not reflect on such issues. By contrast, they often may be deeply prejudiced by an individual dislike of persons or situations and therefore not able to judge neutrally and objectively through careful thinking and taking into account all sides of the matter [6]. Managers are often seen as "systematic, reflective planners" [10, p.15], but end up in being disorganized, superficial and inefficient [10]. This is something what we have many times experienced in reality, with our superiors and – and quite often with ourselves as well. Where does the problem lie?

Many times theories are well- known, but their practical application fails in the transformation to the real-life situation due to changed environment, resistance of involved staff, lack of flexibility or simply frustration and inabilities of the managers to implement the theories into a suitable practical way. Moreover, many managers may not set their priorities right and get entangled in petty issues, which are not beneficial to anybody [6]. Another problem is the fact that many managers often seem to lack basic skills like fundamental knowledge, leadership skills and understanding of their business as well as their key assets, their staff. They have been moved into positions they cannot fill out and fail in the medium to the longer term thus leading to a major damage of their organization [6]. Rationality models have been seen as the solution for those pressing issues, but they also do not fulfill their purpose in reality, due to major problems with measurement of values. The steps in the rationality model like information gathering, identification of all suitable options, review of the respective consequences and their relation to values with finally choosing the best option [3] are in general good and convenient steps. Nevertheless, they had been heavily disputed. Theories often tried to understand even the phenomenon of innovation [11] and improvisation [13] but did not really grab it. It does not seem to help in reality, to use the overloaded theories with their failed trials to understand, define and explain issues that should be better done from personal intuition and feeling [6]. Only veterinary practitioners or veterinary practice managers with critical-thinking abilities will be competent to cope with the ever-changing situations and expectations and decide for the best of their veterinary practices and hospitals. So what is the solution for all these issues that are negatively impacting the business?

5.3. PRACTICAL APPLICATION OF THEORIES

The best way to get a benefit out of theories is to break them down to their basic idea and to evaluate if this is suitable for the veterinary practice. All the newly developed terms are just to make a name for the authors but not to make sense out of them. But how can we apply the basics in a way that is works in veterinary practice? To get started it is best to have a very down-to-earth approach. The basic idea or the nucleus of a theory has to be reviewed in the context of the business idea. Actually, it does not matter which theory it is and who developed it. It matters only if the basic part of the theory helps in improving the business and adds an additional competitive advantage to it. If the basic part of the theory is suitable, then understanding about its practical use and benefit needs to come next. It may help to try to integrate the theoretical idea in the business in a kind of pilot project, test it and then evaluate it to see the difference before and after the implementation. For this purpose, a diagram has been developed to demonstrate this thinking process [6]. But where do we start when looking at our business process, strategy and business planning? Let's get started with planning of the veterinary practice and identify the business idea.

5.4. THE BUSINESS IDEA

The business idea of the veterinary practice is the first step towards developing the business plan. Do you plan to set up a small or large animal practice? Are you satisfied to have a sole ownership practice just for normal routine work or do you want to grow the veterinary practice over time? Do you want to focus on one market segments only e.g. feline or equine or do you look for a modular practice design with several pillars to protect you in difficult economic times? This might include the combination of the veterinary practice with integrated pet shop and boarding facilities. The distinct competencies for the business idea with subsequent business planning are specialized knowledge of the local market, definite professional knowledge in new service areas like wellness and homeopathy apart from conservative treatment as well as the understanding of the potential customers needs. This leads to the competitive advantage of the new veterinary practice compared to the already established veterinary clinics [7].

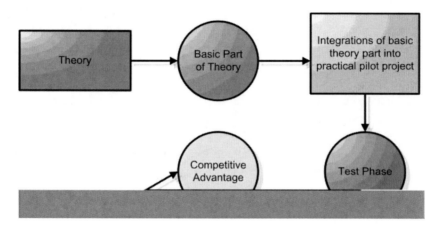

Figure 5.1. Application of theories in practice [6].

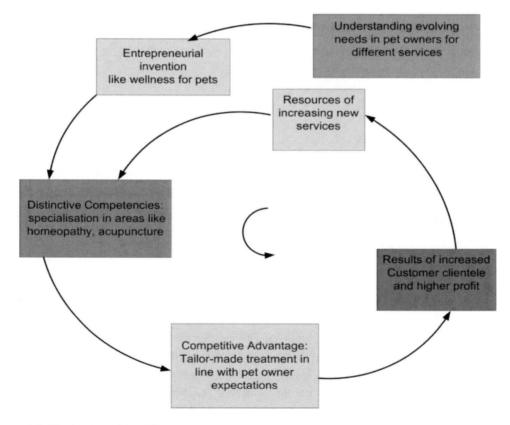

Figure 5.2. The business idea [7].

Following the clear business idea, one of the most important start activities for the setting up of a veterinary practice is to think about everything that is important to the new practice. Those major factors like general, financial and operational issues can be taken into consideration in a brainstorming model. Such a brainstorming model is a highly effective tool for decision-making and a great step towards working on a veterinary practice business plan.

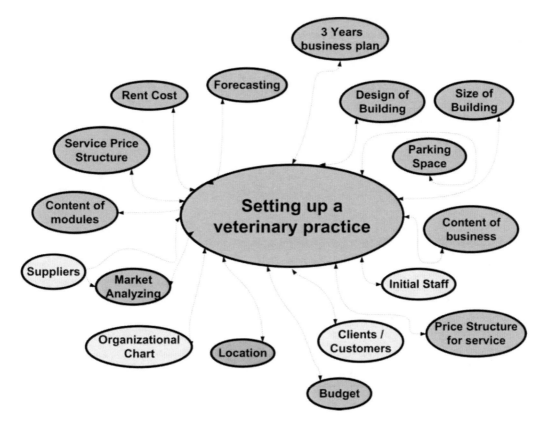

Figure 5.3. Brainstorming model for setting up a veterinary practice [7].

5.5. GETTING STARTED WITH BUSINESS PLANNING

Sometimes veterinary practitioners ask themselves why they should make a business plan. The answer is easy: business planning is essential for every kind of business, including veterinary practices as it reviews the financial commitment, time and resources required for a successful business. Therefore, the advantages of business planning are manifold. They include a realistic assessment of resources like time, money [2] and staff. Moreover, the setting up of the business plan forces the veterinary practitioner to put clearly the steps in order and to establish measurable milestones that have to be achieved [2]. This is often not very easy for veterinary practitioners as they are not used to be confronted with such way of business thinking and working.

Many veterinarians find it difficult to establish a complete business plan and sometimes do not fully understand the importance of the business plan for the future success of their veterinary practice. A well-prepared business plan can help in obtaining easier financial aid from banks as bankers recognize that the loan will be invested in a safe and well structured project. Moreover, business planning leads to have a closer look at important issues like amount of investment and cash flow.

Often underestimated by new practice owners, cash flow can prove to be of utmost importance in the survival of the veterinary practice. If the cash flow is estimated at a too low level, the newly opened veterinary practice may find itself in the situation that the cash money runs out. In the worst case, this lack of cash money may lead to the inability to pay bills and subsequent bankruptcy. Business plans cover all significant topics like mission, success keys and summaries of the veterinary practice as company, services, market's analysis as well as the strategy.

Management plans and especially the highly important financial plans are included in a well-designed business plan, too. Before starting to write up the business plan, a profound research has to be done to understand clearly the market and competitor's situation for the veterinary practice.

This is vital for the success of the new practice as it will directly influence its income structure. A good way to plan for all eventualities is the setting up of three scenarios, the optimistic scenario, the easy to achieve and the pessimistic scenario [2].

This helps the new practice owner to be readily prepared for all different situations that veterinary practice may face especially in the first years. Some points should be avoided in a good business plan. They include setting unrealistic long-term projections and goals and overly optimistic assumptions and calculations.

A business plan should always be better planned on the conservative side with special emphasis on capital investments, cash flow, timelines as well as service income and profits. Difficult language and veterinary specific terminology should be avoided. Moreover, the veterinary practitioner or practice manager should not forget to revisit the business plan regularly and update it according to the current situation.

This will lead to a full preparedness of the veterinary practice even in difficult economic times and helps to foresee and prevent economic troubles of the practice at an early stage.

Nowadays, readymade business plans are available on the internet and solid business plan software packages for veterinary practices can be bought, which provide a great help in structuring the business plan, especially for inexperienced veterinary practitioners.

5.6. GETTING STARTED WITH MAKING STRATEGY

The first point when getting started with making strategy is to clearly identify for which practice the strategy will be developed. Is it the individual veterinary practice or is it for a larger veterinary hospital with a conglomerate of several branches that might be performing different services?

The latter might sometimes come into a situation that leads to the urgent need for developing a new strategy outline following changes in its business or even sub strategies for its special branches.

5.6.1. Brainstorming Process

5.6.1.1. Strategy Team and Time Frame

Forming the first strategy or looking for a new strategy for the veterinary practice is not an easy task that can be done within a few minutes only. It has to be thoroughly worked through several important questions to understand fully and plan where the veterinary practice is heading to. For this purpose, it is useful to implement a strategy making team that consists of the most important members of the future or existing veterinary practice. This may include e.g. the veterinary practitioner who is the practice owner, practice owner partner, practice manager, assistant veterinarian and head nurse. Each team member gets one of the following special roles assigned:

- Opinion former
- Idea generator
- Sit back and wait and see before jumping
- Facilitator
- Client

Depending on the number of team members, some members can hold double functions like facilitator and client in the same time [6]. The idea of this role play is to brainstorm and to generate ideas from different points of view. The identification of the time horizon follows as the next step. A good time line for the time horizon is three years. A two-year period would not be long enough whereas a five-year period would be too lengthy regarding the immense changes ahead [6].

5.6.1.2. Issues and Interrelations

The identification of veterinary practice issue and interrelations are the next point. All topics that relate to this point are brainstormed and put it a diagram. The diagram may contain as many topics as required. They can include issues like 'new services to generate more income', 'quality of work dropping down', 'keeping costs low', 'cutting costs', 'increase staff training', 'increase loyal customer clientele' etc. As a sample, a simplified diagram is shown below to explain how to compose such a diagram.

5.6.1.3. Goals and Distinctive Competencies

Goals

From the previous brainstorming exercise, several clusters can be put together that form emerging goals. Those goals are vital for the strategy forming.

Goals can be either positive or negative. Negative goals may lead to major negative impact on the veterinary practice business and should be regarded with extra caution. They can be transformed to positive goals when being formulated in a more favorable way and linked to positive goals [1].

Goals can be differentiated into core goals that are essential to the business and facilitative goals that have main focus on the internal support functions [1] of the veterinary practice, e.g. software and IT functions.

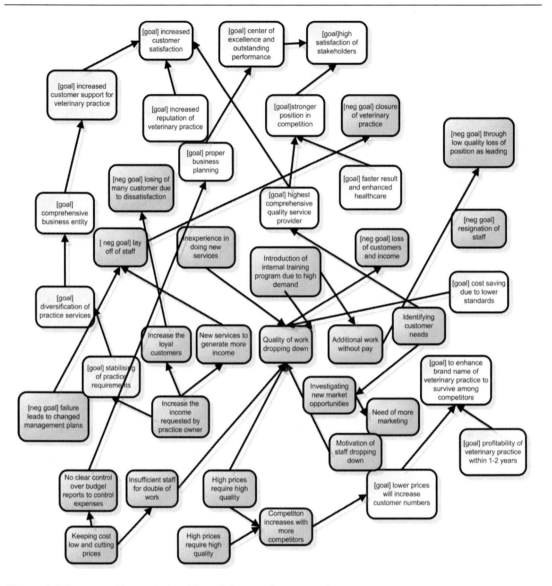

Figure 5.4. Issues and interrelationships of the veterinary practice.

Competencies and Distinctive Competencies

Competencies are the drivers that differentiate the veterinary practice from other veterinary practices. Especially, the core competencies will lead to the competitive advantage of the business compared to other veterinary practices.

Competencies may include points like expert medical team, advanced machinery and equipments, wide customer range compared to other competitors, building of customer trust, excellent reputation of veterinarians and veterinary practice. Long term expertise in a special veterinary discipline may be regarded as core competency of the veterinary practice. When putting these competencies together, the diagram will look as follows:

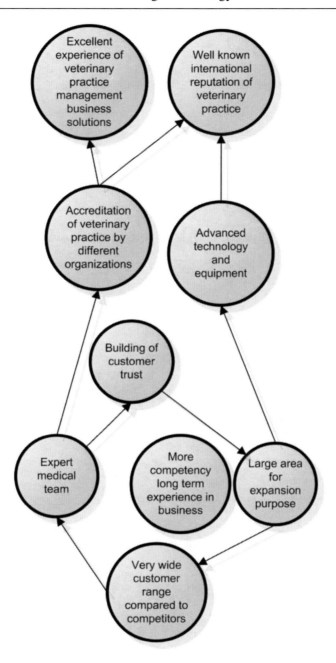

Figure 5.5. Competencies and distinctive competencies diagram.

Linking Goals with Competencies

Some competencies do have a connection to the previously established goals. However, not all competencies or even the core competency will be linked to goal, which is normal and does not cause a problem for the strategy formulation. It is possible to establish revised goals. Goals are linked with competencies as shown below.

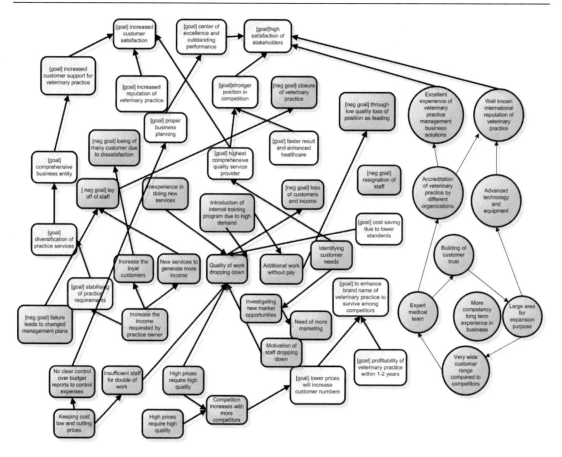

Figure 5.6. Linking goals with competencies.

5.6.2. Statement of Strategic Intent

All previous exercises lead to the formulation of the statement of strategic intent. It includes the following 3 levels:

There is the expectation that:

Highest comprehensive quality service provider

- Enhanced reputation of veterinary practice
- Increase the reasons to become a new customer
- Increased customer satisfaction
- High satisfaction of stakeholders

These levels of expectation can be supported by:

- Long-time experience in business
- Well-known reputation of veterinary practice and team
- Excellent experience of veterinary practice management for business solutions

And require:

- Increase in income requested by practice owner
- New services to generate more income

Without compromising:

- Quality of work dropping down
- Additional work without pay

> The Happy Veterinary Practice will seek the position of HIGHEST COMPREHENSIVE QUALITY SERVICE PROVIDER. This position will enhance its own reputation. This level of reputed service providing will increase the reasons to become a new customer and lead to increased customer satisfaction and high satisfaction of stakeholders.
>
> We will extend our long-time experience in business. Significantly, we aim at increasing our well-known reputation of the veterinary practice and its team. We will widen the excellent experience of veterinary practice management for business solutions.
>
> We recognize that in order to achieve these circumstances, we must increase our income as requested by the practice owner and therefore, introduce new services to generate more income. This needs to be done without compromising the quality of work and by rewarding additional work.

5.7. FINANCIAL PLANNING - START UP COSTS

Now we know what we want to be and what we like to achieve with the new veterinary practice. But how much will the new veterinary practice cost? For each business, the accurate estimations of required set up costs are essential and are often underestimated thus leading to undercapitalization and subsequent financial problems of the new business [5]. Many small businesses fail due to lack of sufficient capital and cash flow to keep the business running until the break even or a profit is reached [9]. Startup costs of veterinary practices have to be established like in any other small business. They can be quite considerable depending of its size and equipments. Startup costs include equipment, furniture, computer hardware and software, legal but also rent and insurances. A list of startup requirements has been set up below. Therefore, good planning is essential especially as a newly opened business might usually not be profitable in the first year of existence.

Savings should make up at least 30-50% of the startup costs with the rest of the required money being borrowed. Apart from own savings, money can be raised from family members and friends which might get easy access to the required funds, but in the same time can put pressure on the relationships. Bank loans are the frequently used alternative of borrowing money. It is important to get the best deals for interest rates. Hence, it is essential to compare loan offers of several banks. Investments can be provided from outside investors as well. This possibility implies that full control over the business will no longer be in the hands of the practice owner. However, it has to be made clear that no bank will invest in a new business which is lacking a thorough business plan. The better the business plan, the better the chances to get loans approved by banks. Bankers want to see that the new business has a chance to survive in highly competitive markets, and they are investing in a long-term profitable capital. They will not take the risk to lend money in a business that is destined to fail due to poor business and financial planning. Startup costs do not only include the costs of assets like equipment and machinery, but also rents, salaries, which are the very important points in terms of cash flow forecasts. First, the working capital has to be identified, which is "the difference between current assets and current liabilities. This total is known as net current assets." [8, p.170]. The second important part is the cash budget which covers working capital that has to be paid out of the pocket for incurring expenses. In general, startup costs have to include initial expenses, monthly money reserves, start up inventory and other expenses.

Table 5.1. Startup costs [modified from 9]

Initial expenses	Monthly money reserves	Other expenses
Legal costs	Salary of business owner	Fixtures
Stationary	Salaries of employees	Equipment
Website costs	Taxes	Signage
Rent deposits	Rent	
Phones	Marketing	
Bank account set up fees	Utilities	
Computers	Phone/mobile costs	
Insurances	Internet	
Construction costs	Insurance	
Installation costs	Car payments, maintenance	
	Bank charges	

The startup of a veterinary practice does not only have general costs but also specific requirements. They range from equipments over furniture to kennels. An example of how to set up startup costs is shown in the table below.

Table 5.2. Sample startup costs requirements for veterinary practices

Happy Veterinary Practice Start-up expenses	
Equipments Medical/Surgical	$ 70,000
Equipment Laboratory	$ 35,000
Equipment Kennel	$ 8,000
Practice furniture	$ 8,000
Vehicle	$ 25,000
Stationary	$ 2,000
Rent	$ 4,000
Insurance	$ 3,000
Legal	$ 3,000
Computer software	$ 2,000
Computer hardware	$ 10,000
Total start-up expenses	$170,000
Start- up assets	
Cash required	$ 30,000
Other current assets	$ 0
Long-term assets	$ 90,000
Total assets	$120,000
Total requirements	*$290,000*

Start up costs can be calculated in the following equation [7]:

Start up costs=Total initial expenses + (total monthly expenses x 3-6 months)
+ start up inventory + other expenses

Some veterinary practice startup costs can be saved when purchasing a second-hand equipment and material in very good condition from e.g. practice closures. Refurbished items can save money at the beginning, too. Another way of cost saving in a good way is the use of heavy-duty kitchen furniture instead of very expensive practice furniture, which is available in specialized kitchen furniture shops. They can last for many years and look like practice furniture.

5.8. SAMPLE BUSINESS PLAN

How do we know what we want and how much it will cost us? This is the time to go ahead and start getting it with the help of a well-founded business plan. For this purpose, a sample business plan has been created to serve as a step-by-step tool box. The sample business plan provides information about the structure of the business plan and its components in detailed levels. It is a systematic assessment of all factors that are critically impacting the veterinary practice's goals. Well designed charts and tables are essential to visualize the forecasts and help in interpreting them. In the sample business plan, not all charts and tables have been included as most of them were explained in detail in other chapters of this book already. Specific comments to each section in the sample business plan will highlight possible pitfalls and areas where special caution needs to be applied.

5.8.1. Executive Summary

Veterinary Practice Business Plan

Happy Veterinary Practice, Happytown

Happytown has a population of 30,000 middle-income residents with small adjacent villages that amount to another 5,000 residents. Many residents are either young families with children and pets and elderly people with mainly cats and dogs. The adjacent villages include farms with cattle and horses. The next biggest city is 30 minutes away by car. The only existing veterinary practice is a practice that offers exclusively basic treatment for pets and does not have surgical facilities.

Happy Veterinary Practice will be owned and run by John Bond DVM and Jenny Smith DVM. Both have 10-year professional experiences with John specializing in surgery, advanced imaging and large animal medicine and Jenny having vast experience in small animal medicine with board certification in veterinary dentistry and homeopathy. Although both have not worked in Happytown, Jenny is born in Happytown and has many friends and family members here. More than 70 friends and acquaintances are already waiting for the Happy Veterinary Practice to open in order to bring their pets as new customers. Through John's and Jenny's specializations, a large variety of services can be offered to a client base that did previously not have access to these services. An investment capital of 120,000 US$ exists in savings of John and Jenny.

Tip:

The executive summary of a business plan should include information about the proposed business, market, management and may also contain funding. The summary comes first but is usually written last as this helps to gather all required information. Moreover, while working through the complete business plan, ideas and vision become much clearer when being put in the overall and especially the financial context.

5.8.1.1. Objectives

Our objectives are as follows:

1) To complete practice facility's renovation by August 1st, 2011
2) To solicit new customers among acquaintances by October 1st, 2011 with target penetration of 80-90%
3) To increase customer base with 600 visits per month by December 31st, 2011 with target penetration of 25-35%
4) To open a referral service for veterinary dentistry until December 31st, 2011

Tip:
Objectives help to outline clearly for potential investors the plan ahead soon and to establish milestones that are achievable.

5.8.1.2. Mission

Our goals are to provide the highest standard veterinary medicine to pets and large animals by offering a latest state-of-the-art range of veterinary services. Our compassionate and caring healthcare for animals is strengthened by the strong relationship of our animal patients and their owners with our dedicated veterinary team. Our mission is to make those services affordable for our customers without compromising their quality.

Tip:
Mission statements should be concise and clearly formulated. It can be helpful to include the relationship between the animals and their owners and the veterinary team in the mission statement.

5.8.1.3. Keys to Success

The keys to success are:

1) Existing investment capital
2) Excellent professional experience in a wide range of services and animal species
3) Dedicated and individualized approach to each patient
4) Low staffing costs
5) Long standing contacts to potential customer clientele

> Tip:
> It is helpful to include tangible key success factors and to identify real factors instead of writing just general factors.

5.8.2. Company Summary

Happy Veterinary Practice will provide a full range of veterinary services to pets and large animals as well as referral services in veterinary dentistry. It will be located in Happytown.

> Tip:
> Company summary should include the location and main services that the veterinary practice provides to its customers.

5.8.2.1. Company Ownership

John Bond, DVM, and Jenny Smith, DVM, are both licensed doctors of veterinary medicine. They are the co-owners of Happy Veterinary Practice.

> Tip:
> Short and concise. It may be helpful to add the fact that the owners are licensed veterinarians.

5.8.2.2. Startup Summary

The primary staff of Happy Veterinary Practice will be John Bond and Jenny Smith, supported by Susan Hyde as the head nurse who worked previously with John. Melissa Green will be hired as the receptionist cum laboratory technician, the same position that she held when working in the same practice as Jenny in the past. Happy Veterinary Practice startup costs include the investment of 120,000 US$ by John and Jenny. A bank loan of 100,000 US$ will be secured by them. The startup costs include the medical, surgery and laboratory machinery and equipment as well as the renovation and remodeling of the practice facilities of 40,000 US$.

> Tip:
> It can be very useful to highlight the initial expenses, assets, investments and loans in a chart as well as to integrate startup costs. They are mentioned in detail in the chapter 9 "Finance, Financial Accounting and Financial Management" in this book.

5.8.2.3. Location and Facilities

Happy Veterinary Practice will be located in a 160 m^2 rented ground floor flat in a commercial premise the Central Street of Happytown. Central Street is the main street, easily accessible by all areas of Happytown and with high-traffic frequency. Parking is allocated to this premise directly in front of the building.

> Tip:
> It is useful to mention the traffic frequency of the street where the practice is located as well as the parking situation.

5.8.3. Services

Happy Veterinary Practice will provide a full range of services with latest technological equipments and professional expertise.

5.8.3.1. Service Offering

The service offering of Happy Veterinary Practice will include:

1) Small animals internal medicine
2) Large and equine internal medicine
3) Soft tissue and orthopedic surgery
4) Dentistry
5) Alternative medicine and homeopathy
6) Diagnostic imaging
7) Laboratory services
8) Reproductive services
9) Home visits

> Tip:
> List the important services but not basic services like general examination or vaccinations as they are routine services for every veterinary practice and do not show special expertise. It is also possible to make one small sentence for each service.

5.8.3.2. Technology

Happy Veterinary Practice will use Happy vet Software, which is a comprehensive veterinary hospital management software, including payroll, inventory and accounting module. The website will be connected to the software and enabled for electronic payments. Latest technology will be also introduced by installing a digital X-ray and ultrasound with color doppler.

5.8.4. Market and Competitor Analysis Summary

Happy Veterinary Practice is located centrally in the middle of Happytown within reach of 10-15 minutes by car from all different areas. The adjacent villages are within reach of maximum 20 car minutes. Currently veterinary services are underrepresented in Happytown with only one existing veterinary practice.

The target market for Happy Veterinary Practice is mainly middle-class families with children and elderly people as well as the farmers in the adjacent villages. They all have animals but not sufficient access to veterinary healthcare facilities.

5.8.4.1. Market Segmentation

Our market segmentation scheme divides the market in Happytown in three target groups:

1) Middle-class families: the number of middle-class families has risen in the past three years caused by growing industrialization and opening of new factories and industry plants. This growth will continue, which will lead to further customer potential in newly moved families. This target market is approximate 40% of the market.
2) Elderly people: the number of elderly people is also on the rise with a 35% market share. As grandparents of middle-class families are moving more frequently to Happytown, a higher potential of elderly clients can be expected in the future.
3) Farms around Happytown: the number of cattle farms is decreasing, but the equine population is rising. With a current market share of 25% for cattle and equine owners, the potential of equine as patients will be increasing as one new large riding school and one horse breeding stable are opening end of this year.

> Tip:
> A chart or table can visualize the market analysis and the forecasted projection of a potential customer increase.

5.8.4.2. Competitor Analysis

Happytown has currently only one veterinary practice, Smally Veterinary Clinic. It has been established before 25 years and offers exclusively basic veterinary examinations and treatments like vaccination and deworming as well as neutering. Smally Veterinary Clinic is owned by one veterinary practitioner who is in the same time the only veterinary surgeon in this clinic and holds solely limited two-hour consultation in mornings and afternoons. This clinic does not cover the services that Happy Veterinary Practice intends to offer to the customers.

> Tip:
> It is good to cover weak and strong points of competitors and put them in relation to the new practice.

5.8.5. Strategy and Implementation Summary

The key success factor of Happy Veterinary Practice is the lack of veterinary expertise in Happytown. As Jenny was born in Happytown, she is a familiar face for the population and has many contacts that will be used to enhance the visibility of the practice. Jenny has already informed friends and family about the opening of Happy Veterinary Practice as well as established contacts with the local dog and cat clubs as well as the Horse Riding School.

The location in the middle of the city at the main street is another crucial success factor for Happy Veterinary Practice.

5.8.5.1. Competitive Advantage

The competitive advantage of Happy Veterinary Practice is:

1)   High quality professional expertise
2)   Only veterinary clinic with a full range of services
3)   Central location in the town center
4)   Customers who know Jenny are waiting for practice opening

---

Tip:
The competitive advantage is crucial for getting investments and bank loans but also for the survival of the veterinary clinic. It has to be absolutely clear what is the distinct difference between existing competitors and the own practice.

5.8.5.2. Sales Strategy

The sales strategy of Happy Veterinary Practice is growth in two areas, middle-class and elderly people and referrals from satisfied customers as well as veterinarians in nearby towns. Services will be priced at an average level to match with the expected customer income group.

5.8.5.3. Marketing Strategy

The marketing plan for Happy Veterinary Practice includes an advertisement in the local press as well as listing in the Yellow Pages. Moreover, an interview in the local radio is scheduled already as well as appearances at meetings of the dog and cat clubs. Mailing announcing the opening of Happy Veterinary Practice will be distributed to households of animal owners.

Special flyers will be handed out at supermarkets and major shops. The practice's website will be listed and specially featured in the local community website.

5.8.6. Management Summary

The practice's owners John Bond and Jenny Smith will both equally manage the Happy Veterinary Practice, including daily veterinary and administrative management. The additional two staff will be increased in the second year of operation by one nurse.

5.8.7. Risks/Opportunities

We have identified as greatest risks to our business today the opening of a third veterinary practice in Happytown, another economic recession and the rising unemployment. However, we feel that we are able to overcome these risks because of our high customer satisfaction, excellent expertise and reputation in surgery, homeopathy and veterinary dentistry as well as home visits.

The biggest opportunities that we have identified are becoming a referral center for veterinary dentistry and alternative medicine as well as home visits to elderly pet owners. Moreover, the setting up of new factories and industrial plants provide another big opportunity for growth.

5.8.8. Financial Plan

Happy Veterinary Practice bases its financial plan on cash flow as major source of income. It assumes that veterinary services will remain important to animal's health in the future.

5.8.8.1. Break-Even Analysis
Although the first few months after opening will result in negative financial numbers, the forecast shows that the break-even point will be reached after six months. The estimated break-even point is 35,000 US $ monthly. The fixed costs per month amount to 25,000 US$.

> Tip:
> It is useful to show the break-even chart as well as break even analysis as detailed in the chapter 9 "Finance, Financial Accounting and Financial Management" in this book.

5.8.8.2. Projected Profit And Loss
The first monthly profit is expected in month 6 with a total of 35,000 US$ in year 1. In year 2, the profit will rise to 48,000 US$ and in year 3 to 75,000 US$.

> Tip:
> It is mandatory to provide the Pro Forma Profit and Loss analysis for three years. Moreover, it is good to include a chart for the first year as well as for three years to show the development of projected profit and loss. This is a highly critical forecast for banks and investors.

5.8.8.3. Projected Cash Flow
The lack of cash flow in the first months will be covered by the two practice owners who will use their own funds. The projected cash flow as well as the cash flow chart and cash balance chart are as follows:

> Tip:
> The correct forecast of cash flow is crucial for the survival of the veterinary practice. It is therefore better to be as conservative as possible in the projected cash flow statements. Please refer to chapter 8 "Accounting, Management Accounting and Budgeting" for sample cash flow statements.

5.8.8.4. Projected Balance Sheet
The projected balance sheet for three years is as follows:

> Tip:
> The correct forecast of the balance sheet is important to show the financial position of the veterinary practice at a given time. Please refer to chapter 8 "Accounting, Management Accounting and Budgeting" for sample balance sheet statements.

5.8.8.5. Business Ratios

A variety of important business ratios, including profitability ratio, activity ratio, liquidity ratio, debt ratio and other additional ratios are shown for three years.

> Tip:
> It is useful to show the ratios in a three years' comparison as detailed in chapter 9 "Finance, Financial Accounting and Financial Management" in this book.

5.9. INNOVATION

A veterinary practice is not just a place where all services remain the same over decades. Innovation can be a part of veterinary practices, too. However, what does innovation mean? "The process of innovation is defined as the development and implementation of fresh ideas by people who over time engage in transactions with others within an institutional context." [12, p.139].

When talking about innovation, we are talking about a wide range of innovation, including technical and administrative innovation. Technical innovation includes brand new technologies like minimal invasive surgery and new services. On the other hand, administrative innovation contains the introduction of new policies and procedures, and organizational structure changes [12].

Innovation and implementation of new ideas resemble the product life cycle. In many cases, fresh innovative ideas often come from demanding customers. Therefore, it is important to listen to clients' suggestions and complaints as they may contain the hint to original ideas and a possible introduction of new services. This can add additional value to the veterinary practice.

However, often innovations are met with resistance among staff. Other problems may arise with regard to work processes, and structural or strategic changes [12].

5.9.1. People and Process Problem

Organizations and their staff often focus on keeping already existing work practices instead of integrating new ideas. Another limitation to innovation is also the group thinking and internal conformity as well as organizational constraints.

People act only when confronted direct with problem sources and then are willing to find innovative solutions. Stress leads to vigilance. Therefore, the review and evaluation of options without time restraints are crucial to allow the careful choice of the best decision. Innovation and thus change may trigger fear and resistance among staff [6, 12].

The main problem is to develop the new ideas to a stage that it can be implemented and become routine practice. Therefore, two models of product innovation, the technology-driven model and customer or need-driven model do exist. The problem of part-whole relationship means that often a single part of a new process might function very well, but the combined whole of the process does not give satisfying results.

The usually used linear sequential coupling process for implementation of innovative ideas can lead to mistakes in the end product. Therefore, the simultaneous coupling process is more advisable as it can be considered as a kind of holistic approach [6, 12].

5.9.2. Structural and Strategic Problem

New ideas in the veterinary practice need multidisciplinary approaches and different resources to be transformed in a real life suitable process. The principle of negative feedback leads to set clear and critical limits to innovation. For this reason, the experimentation and selection approach to identify and correct mistakes through double-loop learning is helpful [12]. Keeping a diverse environment in the veterinary practice creates the climate to foster more invention and innovation.

Innovative ideas might result in structural changes of the veterinary practice for their implementation, which require a new infrastructure of the practice itself. The strategic problem of innovation is institutional leadership, which is often required to create a climate and culture suitable and supportive of innovation [6, 12]. It is important to keep the distinctive competence and not to let values emerge in the organization that might act in the opposite way to innovation and structural organizational change [6, 12].

5.9.3. Solution

The solution to these problems is the understanding that innovation is important and may lead to a competitive advantage over the other competing veterinary practices. However, it is the crucial success factor that innovation must be carried and accepted by all staff. In contrast, institutionalization of innovation is not the ultimate aim because it will destroy the spirit and climate to foster for more innovative ideas [6]. Structural changes might be necessary in an progressive veterinary practice, but the general practice structure should not become rigid. All different angles of new ideas have to be reviewed and evaluated according to their advantages and disadvantages. Innovation always has to come from the people and process itself and therefore cannot be imposed on the veterinary personnel. However, it should not be forgotten that creative ideas have a life cycle like the product life cycle and will therefore not stay innovative forever. For this reason innovation has to become an ongoing process to enhance veterinary services and consequently to become the success key and competitive advantage of the veterinary practice.

5.10. CONCLUSION

To conclude, the basic idea of management and strategic theories can be taken and evaluated upon their suitability in the veterinary practice. However, any theory always needs to be adapted to the different situations and their practicalities. It does not help to try to enforce them strictly but to find a way to take the best parts out of them and to implement them in a reasonable and practical way. This will help to create more knowledge businesses and managers that are more able to perform a better job. The aim of this chapter is to introduce the veterinary practitioners to the real business world with strategy and business planning that seems to be often so far away from the veterinary world. However, we as veterinary practitioners should never forget that a veterinary practice is a business, a small enterprise. Our love to animals does not mean that we treat animals exclusively; we also have to take the business part of the veterinary practice into consideration. It does not help to be an excellent veterinarian if the practice goes bankrupt because of missing or wrong business knowledge and understanding. Just to love animals is great but not enough to survive in the business world! Veterinary practitioners have mastered an extremely difficult study and are very well capable of mastering also business planning and strategy.

REFERENCES

[1]   Ackerman, F., Eden.C. and Brown, I. (2005). The practice of making strategy. A step-by-step guide. *Sage publications.* London. Thousand Oaks. New Dehli.

[2]   Ackermann, Lowell (2007). Blackwell's five-minute veterinary practice management consult. Blackwell Publishing. Iowa. USA.

[3]   Cropper, S. Eden, C., Gunn L. and van der Heijden, K. (1990). Principles of rationality. University of Strathclyde MBA Open Learning Materials. In: *Managing, University of Strathclyde Business School.*2006. pp. 62-72.

[4]   Englehart, J. (2001). The marriage between theory and practice. Public Administration Review. 61 (3). pp. 371-374. In: *Managing, University of Strathclyde Business School.*2006. pp.10-13.

[5]   Megginson, W.L., Byrd, M.J. and Megginson, L.C. (2000). Small business management: An entrepreneur's guidebook. 3rd ed. McGraw-Hill. Boston, Madrid, Toronto.

[6]   Muller, M.G. and Abu Aabed, A. (2006). Making strategy. MBA Assignment.University of Strathclyde. *Graduate School of Business.* Glasgow, UK.

[7]   Müller, M.G. and Abu Aabed, A. (2007). Guidelines for setting up a small and medium size enterprise. MBA Thesis, University of Strathclyde. *Graduate School of Business.* Glasgow, UK.

[8]   Nobes, C. (1995). The economist books: Pocket accounting. Penguin Group. Hamondsworth, Middlesex, England.

[9]   Ryan, J.D. and Hiduke, G.P. (2006). Small business: an entrepreneur's business plan. 7th ed. Thompson Soth-Western. Ohio.

[10]   Salaman, G. (1995). Managing. Chapters 3,5&7. Buckingham: Open University Press. In: *Managing, University of Strathclyde Business School.*2006. p.14-25.

[11]   Tushman, M. and Nadler, D. (1986). Organizing for innovation. California Management review, 28(3). pp. 74-92. In: *Managing, University of Strathclyde Business School.*2006. pp.158-172.

[12]   Van den Ven, A. (1986). Central problems in the management of innovation. Management Science, 31(5). pp. 590-607. In: *Managing, University of Strathclyde Business School.*2006. pp.138-156.

[13]   Weick, K. (1998). Improvisation as a mindset for organizational analysis. Organization Science, 9(5). pp. 543-555. In: *Managing, University of Strathclyde Business School.*2006. pp.174-191.

Chapter 6

LOCATION AND PREMISES

ABSTRACT

The location of a veterinary practice is one of the most essential key success factors. Whether the practice is located centrally in the center of a city or on the outskirts in purpose-built premises depends largely on the budget, staff numbers, type of practice, type of services and patient species. A clear analysis of the workflow should be undertaken before finalizing the floor layout as this will save considerable time and increase productivity and profitability. This will also help to determine the allocation of rooms in the front, middle, administrative and support as well as the back area of the veterinary practice. For a well run veterinary practice and hospital, maintenance is an important factor. It has to be planned and budgeted annually and executed according to needs and requirements but also on a routine basis.

6.1. INTRODUCTION

One very important decision for setting up a brand new veterinary practice, buying an existing veterinary practice or constructing a new clinic is the location. This decision depends on the most important factor, the practice owner's budget.

The right location can lead to an increased customer influx as well as generation of new customer clientele. To find the suitable premises can be time consuming, but it is definitely worth it as the veterinary practice will usually remain in these premises for a long time. Moreover, the location of a business has been rated four times more important than outperforming within the market [9].

The choice of the right business location can make a major "difference between success and failure" [3, p.281]. The area around it can be divided in three parts, the primary area which accounts for 75% of the business's income, the secondary area accounting for 20% of the service and product sale and the tertiary area which accounts for only 5% income [8].

Therefore, a business should be located ideally in a primary area with a high population number of potential target clients, providing a stable base of customers. Although the small-business owner such as veterinary practice owner usually does not have too much money to rent a prime location premises, they should invest in this as it is one of the major key factors to success [3, 4, 8].

6.2. LOCATION

The business location should be uncomplicated to find for the clients and in easy reach of public transportation. The veterinary practice should be located in a good area with sufficient potential clientele and access to labor, suppliers and customers' needs to be taken into consideration when choosing the right business location [6].

A suitable area for a veterinary practice should be within 10 minutes [1] to 15 minutes [2] car drive radius. Another measure is ten miles in rural areas and 3 miles in urban areas (Lowell). The average population to support one veterinarian ranges between 4,000 [2] to 10,000 [1, 5] people in the catchment area. Therefore, it is best to research properly the population structure and demographics of the area around the planned practice as this is one of the key success factors for a profitable veterinary practice.

Apart from the catchment area, the suitability of a veterinary practice site depends on various other factors like size, premises condition and parking. The average size of a practice depends on the number of veterinarians and veterinary staff as well as the kind of services offered, and species treated. A clinic with dog boarding facilities needs more space than a clinic with predominantly treatment services. An equine or large animal practice requires much more space than an avian, feline or reptile clinic. Moreover, hospitals with larger outpatient clientele will have fewer space requirements per examination room. They will feature more exam rooms, more short-term holdings and larger treatment spaces but smaller surgical areas and reduced number of long-term hospitalization wards [1]. In contrast, inpatients oriented practices or hospitals require larger consultation rooms, surgeries and specialty areas as well as inpatient wards. Specialty hospitals offering CT scan machines and MRIs have increased space requirements than general veterinary hospitals [1].

In recent years, several large veterinary practices have moved from city centers to the outer industrial areas due to cheaper rents or availability of land for building new practice premises. This can be a good step regarding space, but might be more difficult to reach for pet owners without cars. If the veterinary practice or hospital is intended to become a large referral center, this step might be wise as it offers the possibility to acquire land for a relatively cheaper price and therefore, to get a larger site for a purpose-built veterinary hospital with big parking space. Many referral hospitals are using premises in commercial areas or outside the main city center with good success.

Moreover, for a veterinary practice, enough parking spaces in front of [5] or around the practice in the premises' boundaries [1] is highly important. It is preferable in veterinary hospitals with large boarding facilities to have separate parking facilities for their kennels for drop off and pick up in order to reduce the car traffic flow around the clinic building [1]. In some cities, special requirements regarding parking spaces for commercial premises exist and have to be strictly followed. Therefore, it is advisable to get first information from the municipality regarding particular building and parking requirements before finalizing building plans or premises purchase.

Easy access for clients, delivery vehicles as well as ambulance and civil services is another important factor to select the right practice location. It might not be suitable to establish the veterinary practice in the smallest road in the neighborhood where only one car can drive at a time.

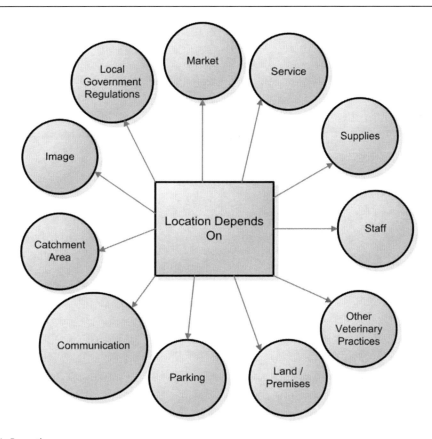

Figure 6.1. Location.

6.3. PREMISES

The premises of the veterinary practice reflect as the visible business card for each veterinary practice. Therefore, great care should be taken to create a positive image through the right premises. The decision to rent or purchase an existing building also depends on available premises. Existing buildings have to be carefully screened for building faults, damages of e.g. roof, water and electricity pipes. Moreover, possible future expansion plans should be taken into consideration with regard to building space and garden space.

The veterinary practice or hospital building should be in good and well-maintained condition and be visible with excellent lights at night. The practice sign board should be illuminated at night [5] to make it simpler for clients with emergencies to find the practice. Ideally, a road sign close to the practice building will help to find the practice easier.

The premises are ideally located at a ground floor level [5] as often large dogs visit the practice. If they are located upstairs, an elevator would be of great help. In case of a double-storey building, the offices should be situated in the upper floor and clinic and kennels in the basement [1]. A new trend is the location of veterinary practices in shopping centers [1], which might bring easy access but can also contribute to increased stress for a sick animal.

A garden or small green area surrounding the premises is useful for dogs as they often prefer to sniff a bit before entering the veterinary practice.

6.4. FLOOR PLAN

The layout of the floor plan has to be well designed to ensure smooth workflow, short walking ways in busy areas and optimal space usage. It depends on the purpose of the veterinary practice, if it is either mainly for consultation and only smaller general routine surgeries, a larger multi-discipline veterinary hospital or a referral practice.

Front Area

The front area consists mainly of the reception and waiting area and examination rooms [1]. It can be extremely useful to create separate waiting areas for dogs and cats in the waiting room. A clearly visible and skillfully designed merchandising area helps to increase sales and to establish an additional source of income. However, expertly designed merchandising areas might require sometimes double or more of the space of the original reception area. Next to the waiting area, the entrance to the examination room(s) is located.

Middle Area

The middle area of the veterinary practice is used for medical and surgical procedures [1]. Close to the examination room, the X-ray room, surgery preparation and surgery room(s) can be found. An intensive care unit for larger practices is helpful and should be located in a quiet but easily reachable part of the premises. The grooming parlor can be located between middle area and administrative area.

Administrative and Support Area

All non medical functions are located in the administrative and support area. This includes the offices, pharmacy, staff toilets, autoclaving and sterilization room, storage room and utilities area. These rooms are helpful as part of a well-structured veterinary practice.

Back Area

The back area includes the hospitalization wards, quarantine area, kennel and cattery. They should have separate external access, especially for drop off and pick up of boarding animals.

The location of the laboratory depends on its size. If the laboratory is just a small laboratory for parasitology and blood hematology and biochemistry with a microscope and few machines, it can be placed in the medical middle area. However, in the case of a fully fledged larger laboratory with microbiology and virology, then it has to be located separately from the medical part between administrative and support area and back area to avoid any contamination and to keep restricted access to the laboratory.

The decision of the most suitable practice or hospital layout depends largely on the workflow. It is advisable to determine the workflow first before allocating areas to special functions. If the way between two rooms is frequently used but too long, valuable time gets lost, which can result in reduced productivity and profitability. Before planning the final architectural layout of the veterinary practice, a workflow diagram will help to determine the location of the individual rooms. In chapter 12 "Operations Management" in this book, a detailed workflow analysis is provided as an example of how to break down workflow analysis and save valuable time. The workflow diagram should be put into context with the expected customer numbers and services.

6.5. MAINTENANCE

Clients have eagle eyes when it comes to the condition of a veterinary practice. They are able to spot small problems like damage in the painting or overgrown grass. From the condition of the premises, they like to draw conclusions about the condition of the practice as well as its professionalism. Even dirty pathways or cigarette stumps in front of the entrance door will be regarded in a negative way. Therefore, it is a must that the practice premises must be always perfectly maintained, no matter if it is the surrounding of the premises or the interior. Even if the veterinary practice owner may think that the maintenance can be postponed for a little while, the client will think that the practice is in a poor economic situation and cannot afford the maintenance. The same applies to machinery and equipment. It does not reflect positively on the veterinary practice when examinations cannot be undertaken because the required equipment is temporarily out of service or completely damaged.

What are the main reasons for maintenance of premises and equipments? The first reason is to have premises in good condition and well functioning equipment, which subsequently leads to a high quality image among the customer clientele [7]. Good working conditions for staff as well as compliance to health and safety regulations [7] are positive aspects of regular maintenance. Accidents caused by damaged flooring or wiring may lead to legal liabilities of the veterinary practice if the causative agents were left unattended. Insurance may even refuse to pay in such cases.

Cost of premises' maintenance is often underestimated but can cause a considerable amount of money. Whether it is the own practice premises or rented ones, maintenance costs have to be included in the annual budget. A yearly plan for regular maintenance is helpful in controlling sometimes spiraling expenses for repairs. However, what should be maintained and how often?

Above table provides average maintenance time requirements. They can be shorter or longer depending on the material or equipment used. Annual maintenance contracts for machinery and equipment can be extremely useful after the warranty has ended. The costs are usually cheaper as having expensive repairs done without a maintenance contract. However, it should be always verified if spare parts are included completely or up to a certain amount in the contract or if those maintenance contracts just cover the maintenance work without providing any routine spare parts. Regular costs are also paintings of facilities as well as equipment maintenance.

For every larger maintenance, it is advisable to get at least three quotations in order to compare the prices. Sometimes major differences can be found, and a comparison of the quotation saves valuable money. Moreover, it is often saving considerable costs when small repairs can be performed by a local maintenance man.

Table 6.1. Veterinary practice maintenance timeframe

Exterior	Interior	Equipment	Infrastructure
Garden: grass cutting bi-weekly	Flooring: every 5 - 10 years	Scales: calibration every 6 months	Drainage: every 12 months
Garden: flowers according to season	Furniture: every 5-10 years	Autoclaves: every 12 months	Electricity and telephone wires: every 3 month
Pathways: cleaning daily, repairs immediately	Fixtures: every 5-10 years	Medical machines e.g. X-Ray, ultrasound: every 12 months	Computer cabling: every 3-6 months
Roof: every 10-15 years	Wall paintings: every 12 months	Laboratory machines: every 3-6months	Water pipes: every 1 month
Windows: cleaning weekly, every 12 months	Signage: every 5-10 years	Kennels and cages: every 10-15 years	Generator: every 1 month
Building: every 12 months	Heating: every 12 months		
Dog outside runs: every 12 months	Air-condition: every 3 months		
Signage: every 12 months	TV system: every 6 months		
Incinerator: every 1 month			

6.6. RENOVATION AND EXPANSION OF THE EXISTING VETERINARY PRACTICE

The renovation of a veterinary practice might be required if an existing building is bought or after a certain period of time. Usually, every five years, a renovation has to be considered [1] that can be of smaller or larger scale. Even painting or landscaping is considered renovation [1].

Typically, a veterinary practice grows so much in five years, that the existing practice facilities are not sufficient anymore, and an expansion needs to be considered. Smaller renovation can be done relatively easily without leading to major disturbances of the daily practice routine. However, larger renovations might disturb the practice workflow considerably. For this reason, the duration and noise intensity of the renovation has to be considered in order to decide whether it makes more sense to do the renovation in a low season time or to close the practice for a short while.

Expansion of existing practice buildings can be difficult to handle during the normal routine work. First of all, the expansion building has to be very well planned with an experienced architect who puts special emphasis on short work disturbances or practice closures.

All required building permits have to be gathered before finalizing the work plan. It might be necessary to change the room allocation temporarily with having e.g. a combined examination room cum surgery if the surgery room gets extended. This might also lead to changes in the workflow and subsequent appointment scheduling.

Moreover, another question is whether the expansion will be funded by the veterinary practice owner or through borrowing a loan from the bank [1]. This budget issue will determine the size of the planned expansion. In case of taking a bank loan, the return on investment has to justify the expenses. This decision depends on the interest rate condition of the bank, whether they are fixed or variable [1].

Building changes either through renovation or expansion lead to increased practice revenue. Even simple renovation work like painting or landscaping results already in improved business profits [1].

6.7. CONCLUSION

The location of the veterinary practice or hospital can be rightly regarded as one of the key factors for business success. The choice of the right location depends largely on the budget but needs careful consideration in any way. The location should be considered to be in the primary areas of the business's income. Furthermore, before choosing the location, the size and type of practice as well as the workflow has to be reviewed before deciding on suitable criteria for the premises. Easy access to the veterinary practice is vital for its success. The patient species as well as the nature of the practice services determine the size of the practice premises and building. Purpose-built facilities and referral centers are nowadays moving to the outskirts of cities and industrial areas due to better land availability and cheaper costs. In contrast, a smaller clinic with elderly patient owners might be much better off in a neighborhood area. For all veterinary practices and hospitals, the sufficient amount of parking space is a must and must be considered as one of the main support factors of the successful veterinary business. The decision of renting or buying a building depends largely on the budget of the practice owner and the availability of suitable practice premises. Before finally deciding this, the floor plan has to be reviewed under the light of work processes, staff numbers and offered services. After the practice is up and running, maintenance becomes an issue that is often underestimated or forgotten. It can be best tackled with inclusion in the annual budget planning. Regular routine maintenance and maintenance contracts help to keep costs under control and to support a smooth operation of the practice. Moreover, it leads to a good image among the customers. The same applies to renovation and building expansions.

REFERENCES

[1]   Ackermann, Lowell (2007). Blackwell's five-minute veterinary practice management consult. *Blackwell Publishing.* Iowa. USA.

[2]   Catanzaro, T.E. (1998). Building the successful veterinary practice: programs and procedures. Wiley-Blackwell.

[3]   Megginson, W.L., Byrd, M.J. and Megginson, L.C. (2000). Small business management: An entrepreneur's guidebook. 3rd ed. McGraw-Hill. Boston, Madrid, Toronto.

[4]   Müller, M.G. and Abu Aabed, A. (2007). Guidelines for setting up a small and medium size enterprise. MBA Thesis, University of Strathclyde. *Graduate School of Business.* Glasgow, UK.

[5]   Ouwerkerk, M. and Schlegel, H. (1997). Erfolgreich Praxisführung für den Tierarzt: Praxismanagament/ Praxismarketing. Hannover. Schlütersche GmbH.

[6]   Ryan, J.D. and Hiduke, G.P. (2006). Small business: an entrepreneur's business plan. 7th ed. Thompson Soth-Western. Ohio.

[7]   Shilcock, M. and Stutchfield, G.(2005). Veterinary practice management. A practical guide. Reprinted, Saunders, Elsevier Ltd. Philadelphia.

[8]   The Entrepreneur Magazine (1999). Small business advisor. 2nd ed. John Entrepreneur Media Inc. Wiley&Sons. New York, Chichester, Weinheim, Brisbane, Singapore, Toronto.

[9]   Viguerie, P., Smit, S. and Baghai, M. (2010). Granularity. Smart choices to grow your business in good times and bad. *Marshall Cavendish Business.* London, UK.

Chapter 7

HUMAN RESOURCES MANAGEMENT

ABSTRACT

Human resources management is one of the most critical factors for the successful veterinary practice. Suitable staff selection and recruitment are a difficult task and require careful consideration of desired character traits and technical skills. After recruitment, individual job descriptions help the new employee to understand clearly the work to be performed as well as the reporting line. However, not only technical skills make a good employee, but also soft skills. Staff competencies are another important factor of how the new employee will fit into the team. Depending on the job profile, competencies can be divided into basic and advanced competencies. Staff has to be motivated to bring high performance. Training and continued professional development will enable veterinary personnel to improve their existing skills and to acquire new ones that are beneficial for the veterinary practice. Performance appraisals can help to track the employees' development and to readjust professional objectives and development plans. Employee satisfaction surveys are a useful tool to assess employees' motivation and work satisfaction.

7.1. INTRODUCTION

Modern business management talks a lot about human resources theories and performance management in order to maximize profits. The often used phrase "An organization does not depend on an individual team member" has resulted in contemptuous treatment of employees and lack of respect of their personal work efforts. However, is this sentence true? It is definitely right that no organization will close because of resignation of team members. However, the more important point is the impact on the organization of a high profile employee's resignation who can be regarded as one of the pillars of an organization. This will not only lead to a vacant position but also to a major loss of work contribution, experience, innovation and creativity as well as dedication, which can result in a major loss to the organization. Often, the consequences of this loss can only be validated fully over the coming years. It is definitely time not just to use human resources theories without looking at the individual, but to put the individual employee in the center of the human resources framework as the main pillar of a strong business development. This applies to all organizations but especially to small high-performance enterprises like veterinary practices where everyone makes a recognizable contribution to the business success.

7.2. Staff Selection and Recruitment

7.2.1. Staff Selection

Veterinary employees have to have certain characteristics that are inevitable for the veterinary practice success. The most important attribute veterinary personnel need to have is commitment, dedication and loyalty. Without these, no veterinary practice can truly exist. The demands on veterinary team members are exceptionally high compared to other professions with regard to long working hours, heavy physical work, and care taking of critically sick animals. Only 100% committed and dedicated team members will be able to cope over an extended period of time. Loyalty is a very critical factor for the veterinary practice as each practice strongly relies on its loyal staff. The stress caused by the work load as well as difficult clients can be immense. Risks from animals whose reaction in case of pain or anxiety cannot be predicted should not be underestimated and require the willingness of employees to take those risks in order to save the animals' lives. Working in the veterinary practice often requires going the extra mile, which needs extremely passionate staff. They are required to be flexible and to react immediately to a change in circumstances, might they be of medical or any other nature. Team work is another prerequisite for good veterinary personnel as each one has to work closely with each other and needs to trust the other blindly. Initiative is another trait that is extremely useful in veterinary staff as often new and challenging solutions have to be found. Veterinary practices are not the suitable work places for people who prefer to work from 8 AM to 5 PM and then go home and forget the work completely. All those requirements have to be clarified to potential employees before recruiting them. If somebody is not prepared to devote everything to the job, then it is wiser not to recruit this person at all. Only if all veterinary staff members are ready to give 100% commitment to the veterinary practice, the practice will be a successful business in all areas.

On the other hand, the employing practice has a responsibility to its staff. This includes foremost respecting them and providing them with a stabile and reliable future and job security. Staff that feels insecure about their future role or employment in the practice will not be concentrating on their work, which will inevitably lead to mistakes. Appropriate salaries are a must if good employees shall be retained. The same applies to a pleasant work atmosphere where positive attitude, humor, motivation and praise reigns and not permanent criticism, disrespect or neglect. Responsibilities have to be correctly distributed, guided and exercised to empower staff and to share the work load. Staff has the expectancy to grow professionally in the veterinary practice and should receive training to improve their professional knowledge and skills. Well trained personnel can lead to added value of the veterinary practice and thus to increased profitability. All this is easier said than done. The veterinary practice owner or manager plays a vital role in the retention of staff through adequate leadership. He is the example that all employees will follow. If he is not living these attributes, he cannot expect his staff to do it. Life is give and take, and this applies to the veterinary practice world, too!

7.2.2. Staff Recruitment

Staff recruitment can be regarded as a critical success factor for veterinary practices. As each practice heavily relies on excellent and competent staff, recruitment requires time, money and efforts to find the most suitable new team member. One of the major issues in the veterinary practice, especially in a newly opened one, is the staff ratio as this is one of the main budget expenses. The number of employees depends on the size of the practice. For a small new practice, one veterinarian with one veterinary technician/nurse will be sufficient for the beginning. However, a receptionist guarding the telephone and making appointments as well as a cleaning staff might be helpful even on a part-time basis. It is helpful to have an experienced or certified veterinary technician/nurse and a trainee veterinary technician/nurse. This does not only save costs but also gives the trainee the chance to learn and benefit from the experience. Moreover, it is a good succession planning tool in case of e.g. maternity leave of the veterinary nurse. For large practices, different staff teams can complement each other like the veterinarian team, nursing team, reception team, administration team and management team. However, this usually works only in a practice with more partners [11].

Recruitment can be done through specialized veterinary magazines and journals. Before recruiting new employees, it has to be clearly identified which qualifications and skills are required for the vacant job profile. The selection criteria have to be clarified at the beginning of the search for a suitable candidate. The advertisements of a vacant position on the veterinary practice's own website have become very popular as this helps to receive CVs from people who are interested in the practice itself and not only looking for a job that can be anywhere. For all positions clear and detailed job descriptions are mandatory. Despite professional skills, a strong love of animals and a good instinct of understanding animals is inevitable for a suitable practice staff. Moreover, veterinary staff is required to be very hard-working and not to refrain from heavy physical work and long working hours.

Table 7.1. Relation between size of practice and employment of new staff
[modified from 2]

Increase in case load	Small animal practice with < 2 veterinarians	Small animal practice with ≥ 2 veterinarians	Average of small animal practice
Longer opening hours	22%	18%	20%
Hire of new vet. Technicians	27%	15%	22%
Hire of new veterinarian	52%	31%	42%

Small animal practice owners prefer to extend their working hours when the caseload is increasing by up to 20% than hiring new staff. They need to have at least an increase of 22% in cases before they decide to recruit one additional veterinary technician. A new veterinarian is employed when the work increases by 42% [2]. However, the size of a practice is one of the major facts regarding employment as small one or two-person practices will hire a new veterinarian only by a large increase of business as large practices employ a new doctor with a much smaller business volume [2].

7.3. JOB DESCRIPTIONS

Clear job descriptions are essential for new staff in order to understand what is expected from them. It can be helpful to use old job descriptions from other or previous staff members and to modify them to suit the vacant position. In some cases, it might be useful to let the staff write their own job descriptions as this enhances ownership and motivation for the new job. However, certain points have to be mentioned always in a proper job description such as:

- Name
- Position
- Department (if existing)
- Main job responsibility
- Other responsibilities
- Location
- Subordinates
- Supervisor
- Educational requirements
- Signature
- Date

Table 7.2. Sample job description

HAPPY VETERINARY PRACTICE	
JOB DESCRIPTION	
Position	Name
Department	
Job summary	
Main job responsibility	
Other responsibilities	
Location	
Supervisor	
Subordinates	
Educational/professional requirements	
Other requirements	
Signature	Date

In modern business, job descriptions contain large amounts of general information about e.g. competencies, which can lead to 3 or four page long job descriptions. The big disadvantage of such a job description is the fact that employees either do not read those unspecific points or read them and forget their real job requirements. Therefore, it does not make much sense to overload the new staff with non essential comments. The best job descriptions are short but clear, precise, comprehensive and easy to understand.

Table 7.3. Sample job description for assistant veterinary surgeon

HAPPY VETERINARY PRACTICE			
JOB DESCRIPTION			
Position	Assistant Veterinary Surgeon	Name	Dr. Jane Bond
DepartmentVeterinary			
Job Summary Provides consultations, treatment and minor surgical procedures for pets under the guidance of the Head Veterinarian. Assists in major surgeries and has special responsibility for in-house patients.			
Main job responsibility Performs routine consultations and examinations Performs X-rays and other required diagnostic methods Performs treatments Performs minor surgeries for pets such as neutering, spaying, injuries and wound closures Applies laboratory results as part of diagnosis. Assists Head Veterinarian in major surgeries Produces relevant reports as per request of the Head Veterinarian Special supervision of in-house patients Conducts the in-house nurse training under supervision of the Head Veterinarian Performs any other duties as assigned by the Head Veterinarian			
Other responsibilities None			
Location In the consultation rooms, surgery and in-patient wards			
Supervisor Head Veterinarian			
Subordinates None			
Educational/professional requirements Master's degree in Veterinary Medicine 1 year experience in small animal practice Experience of neutering and spaying procedures Experience of treating common pet diseases			
Other requirements Good client care skills Good diagnostic knowledge Good surgical knowledge Competent use of computer systems			
Signature		Date	

7.4. STAFF COMPETENCIES

Competency is defined as "the knowledge, skills, ability and behaviors that a person possesses in order to perform tasks correctly and skillfully" [9, p. 175]. This is especially important in a caring and nursing profession like veterinary practices or human hospitals. In those professions, competencies include the ability to perform the job satisfactorily but also to provide effective care to patients [3]. Therefore, professional standards apply not only to medical staff but also veterinary employees. Apart from professional standards, competencies skill checklist have been used with good results. For those personnel which need to improve their competencies, a special training as target learning program can achieve positive results. Competency assessments should be used as a baseline for performance appraisals [3].

Employees' competencies can be divided into soft and hard skills. Soft skills can be regarded as behavioral skills that form part of the emotional intelligence or EQ of a person. Those very individual skills are often associated with the business success. In contrast, hard skills are of technical or administrative nature and form part of the intelligence quotient or IQ. They relate e.g. to occupational requirements and help to get the job done.

7.4.1. Basic Competencies

Important basic soft skill competencies for veterinary staff are:

- Integrity
- Trust
- Loyalty
- Client orientation
- Teamwork
- Process orientation
- Problem solving
- Interpersonal communication

Integrity and Trust
- Acts as a role model for the veterinary practice in demonstrating key work attributes and continually setting higher examples of personal conduct and professionalism
- Intervenes in and solving conflicting situations that impact the veterinary practice from a neutral and unbiased point of view
- Builds awareness about social responsibility

Loyalty
- Builds a culture of loyalty and reliability by acting as role model
- Being able and willing to establish a long-term relationship with veterinary practice even in difficult situations and times
- Commits to veterinary practice to full extent

Client Orientation
- Always works very closely with clients by getting first-hand information and subsequently developing an independent view of their and their animals' needs, improving services and acting in their long-term interest
- Takes time to question and understand the real, underlying needs of clients, beyond those initially expressed
- Brings potential problems to client's attention and identifies possible solutions prior to issues emerging or causing difficulty

Teamwork
- Works constructively with a diverse team members and other people und understands the circumstances when it is appropriate for the needs of the team to come first
- Takes responsibility for creating and maintaining a positive team atmosphere that supports and rewards collaborative behaviors
- Listens carefully and responds constructively to other team members' ideas

Process Orientation
- Organizes people, processes and activities and turn individual tasks into efficient workflow
- Breaks down and simplifies complex work processes and knows how to measure them and uses technology to positively impact quality in standardized and measurable way
- Creates a innovative learning environment leading to the most efficient and effective work processes to create smooth and fast workflow

Problem solving
- Identifies and analyzes problems and weighs their relevance and accuracy
- Generates and evaluates a set of alternative solutions
- Makes recommendations based upon the found solutions

Interpersonal Communication
- Helps bringing out unspoken thoughts, issues and concerns of other team members and clients alike and uses diplomacy and tact while dealing with others
- Writes, presents and explains specific veterinary medical information in a way that clients or less qualified staff understand
- Practices attentive, active and patient listening and accurately reproduces the opinions of others even when disagreeing

7.4.2. Advanced Competencies for Higher-Ranking Staff

Additionally, for higher ranking staff like practice managers, veterinarians, senior veterinary nurses/technicians a more advanced set of soft competencies are required such as:

- Leadership
- Project management
- Adaptability
- Change management
- Developing self
- Developing subordinates

Leadership
- Creates a vision for the veterinary practice and translates it into goals and smaller workable steps
- Communicates the vision and mission of the team and shows commitments to follow them through together with the team
- Understands the full extent of team's capabilities and uses it by making sure that the needs of the team are met by obtaining needed resources and information for them

Project Management
- Has the ability to get together different work processes in a project based on defined work plans and co-ordinates internally as well as externally for its implementation
- Ensures ongoing control, review and monitoring of the progress and functional troubleshooting
- Maintains knowledge schedule and control over quality and budget

Adaptability
- Has the ability to remain flexible during change initiatives
- Thrives in a fast-paced and fast changing work environment
- Remains enthusiastic and keeping a positive work and personal attitude during periods of change even if its outcome is not certain yet

Change Management
- Willingly embraces and actively champions change by communicating the reasons for change and resulting benefits to other staff members
- Creates and supports flexibility by introducing procedures and plans which ensure quick turnaround and encourage flexibility in others
- Presents realities of change and develops together with the team creative and innovative strategies for managing the change

Developing Self
- Stays informed and updated of latest research and emerging trends in veterinary medicine
- Identifies emerging new requirements, methods and techniques and their respective implementation
- Develops new skills and fosters learning by demanding targets or tasks that reinforce learning

Developing Subordinates
- Identifies high potential employees and provides them with opportunities for growth
- Ensures availability and time for developmental resources and measures like training courses for all employees in the same way
- Creates teams with complementary skill sets and promotes the expectation that they will learn from one another

- Mentors employees to set performance goals and expectations, including development and career plans and provides fair, honest and timely feedback

7.5. STAFF MOTIVATION

Many theories have been written about staff motivation starting from Maslow's hierarchy of needs to Taylor's scientific management and Herzberg's two-factor theory [1,7,8]. Maslow describes the basic needs of human beings as the physiological needs like to eat and drink. When these needs are satisfied, people have other needs like security or psychological needs. The longing for security or safety includes stability and protection. The next step in the hierarchy is social needs like belongingness and love. This is followed by esteem needs, which required acknowledgement and recognition. The last step in the hierarchy of needs is the self-actualization where human beings try to develop their potential and achieve for themselves [1, 7, 8].

McGregor describes in his theory negative assumptions of employees as theory X and positive ones as theory Y thus resulting in an entirely different leadership style [1]. Taylor related staff motivation to monetary rewards [1, 7]. Herzberg disagreed with this belief as for him proper working condition and basic salaries are not necessarily satisfying the staff. He regarded those factors as motivators which lead to actual satisfaction of the employees consequently including possible promotion, recognition and increased responsibilities [7]. However, no matter which approach is followed, the equity theory states that "rewards must be seen to be fair compared to what others get for their efforts" [7, p. 61].

What are the positive aspects of motivation in the workplace? Motivated employees will be more productive and produce more and better quality work. Furthermore, they will be less absent and motivation among staff results in increased co-operation and team work as well as openness to change [7, 8]. In addition, motivation leads to less stress-induced sickness and work-related "burn out" syndromes.

How can the above-mentioned theories be translated in the work environment of a veterinary practice in the best possible and satisfying way? Is it really all about pay rises and money?

The Maslow's hierarchy of needs can be also translated in the daily veterinary practice life as some staff will respond more to social needs, and others might prefer the self-actualization step [10]. Employees of a veterinary practice might have very different background, experiences and character, but they must be able to work in a highly motivated team. Motivators for the veterinary staff can be a motivated team leader who knows his team members very well and especially their performance under stress and pressure. Clearly set achievable goals help to engage the team spirit because everybody aims for the same goal. Achieving these goals needs to be rewarded thus enhancing the motivation of the team. Rewards can be both, in a monetary form, e.g. a bonus or in personal development training [8].

An excellent motivator in the veterinary practice is the continued professional development of technical staff and veterinarians alike. Veterinary technicians or nurses can be supported to get a veterinary nursing certification [11], which is nowadays available in many countries as step up of the career ladder. Other very well received motivating rewards might be the promotion of a veterinary nurse to become pet nutrition or behavioral consultant after successfully participating in respective courses [11]. This increase in responsibilities can be tied with a percentage of the income through these services thus increasing the employee's motivation further.

Another way of motivating staff is a well-planned and coordinated marketing strategy which integrates the abilities of the staff in a positive way like preparing dog puppy parties [11].

7.6. STAFF TRAINING

7.6.1. Advantages and Disadvantages

Staff training is an important issue in the veterinary practice. It is vital to have highly qualified personnel as veterinary medicine is advancing at a very fast pace. Therefore, employees have to be updated and trained in new diagnostic and surgical methods. On the other hand, training courses and continued professional education and development pose a budgetary expense and should be spent wisely. The issue of staff retention reflects very strongly in this context. There is no point to provide training for staff who is in the probationary period, to be terminated or expected to resign soon. For other staffs, continued professional education and development is well invested money if the training is done in a field that benefits the veterinary practice. A nurse who attends a nutrition training course and gets certified can help to create additional income through nutrition consultations for clients.

Table 7.4. Advantages and disadvantages of training

Training	
Advantages	Disadvantages
Personal improvement (skills)	Money
Professional improvements (skills, knowledge, techniques)	Time
Expansion of existing services as specialist services	No return on investment if staff is leaving the practice
Introduction of new services	Dissatisfaction and jealousy of other staff
Staff satisfaction and motivation	Rivalry to get training course
Increase in income	Poor staff attitude and unwillingness
Increase in profitability per staff	No interest in training course subject
Increased service quality	
Increased efficiency and effectiveness of staff and work processes	
Multi-tasking of staff	

The same applies for behavioral classes. Keeping all in mind, it comes down to the questions what are the main advantages and disadvantages of training?

As we can clearly see, the advantages of giving training or continued professional education and development to employees outweigh the disadvantages by far. The risk that staff will leave after receiving training courses is always there and can never be ruled out.

However, the impact that well-trained personnel can make in the veterinary practice is far greater than this risk.

7.6.2. Induction Training and on the Job Training

7.6.2.1. Induction Training

The training of employees starts when the newly employed staff enters the veterinary practice for the first time. After arranging the employment formalities with the practice owner or manager, the new job will be outlined in words and in the written job descriptions to clarify what the new employee is supposed to do. Important information such as internal policies and procedures, fire and first aid procedures, health and safety procedures [12] will be given and explained to the new staff. Then it is time for the show around. During this first round through the veterinary practice, the introduction to other team members starts immediately. This can be done either by the practice manager or by the mentor, who is assigned to guide the new employee. This is usually a more senior staff which will take care of the initial on the job training. The practice tour also includes the various departments of the practice as well as general explanations about the most important functions. Induction training programs can range anywhere from 1 or two days up to two weeks if required [12]. The purpose of this induction training is to ease the employment start of the new staff and in the same time to understand their job role in the practice routine. It is also a time for the already employed personnel to learn and evaluate the skill and technique set of the new employees. This helps to understand where specific training has to be given to align the new employee's work methods with the other practice work. The induction period lays the groundwork for the successful integration of the new team member into the existing veterinary practice structure, processes and policies. The better the induction is performed, the smoother the integration of the new employee in the workflow will become.

7.6.2.2. On the Job Training

After the induction, the training on the job begins. This is usually performed by a more experienced or senior staff member who will supervise and mentor the training of the new employee.

The job training can be divided into three kinds, theoretical training, observation and practical training [12]. It depends largely on the characteristic of the new staff which training is the most suitable for him. A very active and hands-on person is better off with practical training whereas the observation-based program works better for cautious, thoughtful and methodical employees [12].

Persons which choose to learn the theoretical skills first and then apply them into practice are suitable candidates for theory-based training and observation programs. Purely theoretical programs are designed for employees who prefer to plan, learn, design and then practice their skills [12].

It is possible to structure the training by giving time frames for each skill that needs to be acquired. This can be e.g. two weeks time for proficient cat spaying or one week for dental ultrasound scaling. However, the prerequisite for such timeline is the caseload and availability of supervision of the different procedures.

7.6.3. Personal Development Plans

A personal development plan should be developed for all employees of the veterinary practice. This includes the objectives of the work as well as required training to achieve these objectives. The personal development plan is not just focused on improving professional skills, but takes technical skills as well as soft skills and competencies into consideration. Training can include intensified in-house training as well as external training in dedicated training facilities. The personal development plan includes in detail the areas where training is required. They have to be linked to the objectives and identified gaps between objectives and competencies. It then states the actions that have to be taken to fill those gaps.

Table 7.5. Sample Personal Development Plan for veterinary surgeon for the year 2012 (reviewed on July 31st, 2012)

Area for development	Actions taken	Timeframe	Courses/training	Date	Completion
Basic Training in ultrasonography	External training course	Till June 31st,2012	Introduction to small animal ultrasonography, Happytown	February 11th+12th, 2012	Yes
	Purchase of ultrasound book			January 25th, 2012	Yes
Advanced Training in ultrasonography	External training course	Till October 31st, 2012	Advanced small animal ultrasonography, Happytown	August 18th+19th, 2012	No
Proficiency in tooth extraction	Job training under supervision	Till March 31st, 2012	Trained in-house under supervision of Dr. Bond	Ongoing in Q1 2012	Yes
Proficiency in emergencies	Long distance training course	Till December31st, 2012	Emergencies and critical care	Ongoing	No
	Job training under supervision	Till December31st, 2012	Trained in-house under supervision of Dr. Smith	Ongoing	No
Negation skills	External training course	Till February 15th, 2012	Negotiating with difficult customers, Management Institute, Smalltown	January 23rd+24th, 2012	Yes

Actions can be done in the form of self-study, e.g. through long distance training course or professional books, coaching, on the job training under supervision of a more experienced staff member as well as attending external workshops or training courses. The timeframe serves as a line for prioritization as urgent gaps need to be filled first followed by less important gaps. A clear date for completion like e.g. six months has to set to underline the importance of fast, comprehensive and efficient learning.

7.6.3.1. Residential Training Courses

Nowadays, the need for veterinary specialization is tremendously increasing. This does not only help the professional expertise of veterinary surgeons, but also add value and the competitive advantage to the veterinary practice. In some areas, especially in surgery and advanced diagnostic methods like ultrasound and endoscopy, attendance of training courses is mandatory to get practical firsthand experience.

For example, in Europe, the European School for Advanced Veterinary Studies offers a variety of specialist courses with usually 3-10 day residencies. Part of the program can then be performed online. Their courses include [6]:

- Behavioral Medicine
- Cardiology
- Dentistry
- Dermatology
- Diagnostic Imaging and Ultrasonography
- Emergency and Critical Care
- Endoscopy
- Exotic Pets
- Feline Medicine
- Surgery
- Soft Tissue Surgery
- Internal Medicine
- Neurology
- Neurosurgery
- Ophthalmology
- Ophthalmic Surgery
- Radiology
- Small Animal Reproduction
- Equine Medicine

Another extraordinary range of highly practical two-day intensive training seminars is provided by private companies like Eickemeyer Veterinary Equipments Inc. in Germany, who claims to be Europe's largest veterinary training centre [5]. Taught by international veterinary specialists, these courses provide excellent value for money and can bring a good return on invested course fees.

Another advantage is that they can be implemented immediately in the daily practice life and add additional value to the practice.

7.6.3.2. Long Distance Veterinary Training Courses

Nowadays, a large selection of excellent online courses for continued professional education and development are available on the internet and can support staff training without having lost working days. Special nursing courses are mainly intended for veterinary support staff like veterinary technicians or nurses or people waiting for their admission at veterinary schools. Most of those courses are accredited and offer certificates or diplomas after successful completion, which takes as an average between several months and up to three years. Some of those special long distance courses are offered for employees who want to get certified as:

- Veterinary assistant
- Veterinary technician
- Veterinary Technology Associate in Science

Furthermore, the reception personnel have a range of education courses available that are completely long distances learning. Among them are:

- Veterinary receptionist
- Medical administrative assistant
- Medical coding and billing

For practice managers, veterinarians or veterinary nurses who plan to enter the administrative side of the practice, a Master of Business Administration (MBA) can be strongly recommended. Several excellent universities offer long distance MBAs or Masters in hospital / public health management, which are highly beneficial in the veterinary practice administration and management work.

The Certificate in Veterinary Practice Management has been introduced in UK 10 years ago with an average of four graduates annually [12].

In addition, online veterinary education includes long distance training courses for various animal species or general animal health care at colleges in USA, Australia and UK.

Among them is The Centre for Veterinary Education of the University of Sydney that also offers a large variety of long distance learning course for veterinarians such as [4]:

- Avian Medicine
- Behavioral Medicine
- Cardiorespiratory Medicine
- Dermatology
- Diagnostic Imaging
- Emergency Medicine
- Feline Medicine
- Internal Medicine
- Medical Oncology
- Ophthalmology
- Sonology
- Surgery
- Equine Reproduction
- Ruminant Nutrition

General courses about a variety of various animal species and alternative medicine exist as online or long distance learning that covers information for veterinary support staff as well as veterinarians. Their duration can take anytime between a few hours up to several months.

The decision, whether to attend residential or long distance courses depend on the accreditation, time and money as well as the topic. Accreditation of courses is a must if the course is intended for professional career development and not just for general knowledge enhancement. The right course should be weighted carefully to achieve the maximum benefit from continued professional education.

Table 7.6. Long distance courses for various animal species

Canine/Feline	Equine	Fish	Animals	Alternative Medicine
Canine science	Equine science	Fish biology	Animal care	Veterinary homeopathy
Dog grooming	Equine studies	Aquarium and fish keeping	Animal health	Animal physiotherapy
Dog obedience trainer/instructor	Equine energy therapy	Marine biology	Animal science	Energy healing for animals
Feline science	Equine business management		Animal communication	Healing for companion animals
	Stable management		Animal behavior	
			Animal nutrition	
			Zoology	
			Ornithology	
			Ecology	

7.6.3.3. Review of Personal Development Plans

Personal development plans have to be periodically reviewed to be beneficial for staff and practice owners or managers alike. They include evaluation of the attended course or training session. The subjective outcome for the participating staff as well as the more objective information by the supervisor of the application of the newly learnt skills in the daily routine work should be captured in an evaluation form. A quantitative evaluation includes the cost of the training and its outcome as increased productivity or profit [12]. Attendance rates have to be reviewed and assessed. In case of low attendance rates of e.g. internal training courses, the reasons for it have to the identified and if possible taken into consideration for scheduling future in-house training [12].

For each employee, the personal development plan can be combined with the feedback or review forms of the training including all actions taken, certificates and evaluation forms. In some countries, continued professional development cards are used by all veterinary staff.

The evaluation of professional and personal improvement through training and courses will then be further evaluated in the performance appraisal. The objectives stated in the appraisal form can be adapted in the next review if some knowledge gaps have been closed but other might have become evident over the course of time.

The general evaluation of training impact on the veterinary practice and not just the individual should be undertaken to pave the way for future training plans and their readjustment. Training costs have to remain within the allocated budget. Training courses have to be distributed equally among staff even if different topics are taught. Often special equipments or resources might be necessary to implement the learnt skills into practice, which have to be provided. Otherwise the learnt skills and techniques will become forgotten, and this results in complete waste of money and time.

7.7. PERFORMANCE APPRAISALS

Performance appraisals are performed to assess the performance of employees with regard to given objectives. This is usually done on an annual basis with the possibility to conducting quarterly or half yearly appraisals. Their result will affect the personal development plan for each staff. Appraisals should form the baseline for promotions or salary increases. Large formal appraisals like 360° feedback appraisals might be good in business companies, but might not achieve the expected results in a veterinary practice with few staffs only. However, smaller-scale performance appraisals can be beneficial for any size of veterinary practice.

Table 7.7. Sample performance appraisal for a newly employed assistant veterinary nurse

Performance Appraisal for 2012 For Ms. Margaret Smith Assistant Veterinary Nurse	Excellent	Good	Average	Poor
1.Objectives				
• Supports head nurse in in-patients care				
• Supports veterinarian during consultation				
• Gains proficient knowledge of sterilization of instruments				
• Gains proficient knowledge of pet nutrition				
2. Basic Competencies				
Integrity and Trust				
• Acts as role model for personal and professional conduct				
Loyalty				
• Fully committed				
Client Orientation				
Works closely with clients				
Teamwork				
• Works constructively with a diverse team members				
Process Orientation				
• Simplifies work processes				
Problem solving				
• Identifies and analyzes problems				
Interpersonal communication				
• Helps bringing out unspoken thoughts, issues and concerns				
4. Technical Skills				
• Recognizing condition of sick animals				
• Demonstrating nursing care skills				
• Demonstrating instrument sterilization skills				

Performance Appraisal for 2012 For Ms. Margaret Smith Assistant Veterinary Nurse	Excellent	Good	Average	Poor
• Supports in monitoring of in-patient care				
5. Personal Development				
• Knowledge of veterinary nursing/assistant work				
• Knowledge of animal nutrition				
• Knowledge of veterinary instruments and their sterilization				
Appraiser (name and signature)				
Appraisee (name and signature)				

Performance appraisals consist of different sections. They include objectives, basic and advanced competencies, technical skills and personal development. All performance appraisals have to be discussed among the appraiser and the appraisee and signed off by both. Performance appraisals should never be biased and conducted in an honest and fair way. Each employee should get clear objective for each calendar year to know what is expected from him throughout the year. Appraisals can only work if employees know what they are supposed to do.

In contrast to junior position, higher-ranking staff members have more requirements including advanced competencies. Therefore, their performance appraisal should be with much more in-depth details as they are supposed to hold a high ranking position or to take over a leading position in their respective fields in the veterinary practice hierarchy.

Table 7.8. Sample performance appraisal for veterinary surgeon

Performance Appraisal for 2012 For Dr. Jane Bond Veterinary Surgeon	Excellent	Good	Average	Poor
1.Objectives				
• Ensures independent handling of night duties and emergencies				
• Gains proficient knowledge of ophthalmic examinations				
• Gains proficient knowledge of ultrasound examinations				
• Gains proficient knowledge of major surgeries				
2. Basic Competencies				
Integrity and Trust				
• Acts as role model for personal and professional conduct				
• Intervenes in conflicts				
• Solves conflicts				
Loyalty				
• Acts as role model for loyalty and reliability				
• Establishes long-term relationships				
• Fully committed				
Client Orientation				
• Works closely with clients				
• Understands real need of clients				
• Provides solutions to clients in case of problems				

Table 7.8. (Continued)

Performance Appraisal for 2012 For Dr. Jane Bond Veterinary Surgeon	Excellent	Good	Average	Poor
Teamwork				
• Works constructively with a diverse team members				
• Creates positive team atmosphere				
• Listens and responds to team members' ideas				
Process Orientation				
• Organizes people and processes				
• Breaks down and simplifies complex work processes				
• Creates a innovative learning environment				
Problem solving				
• Identifies and analyzes problems				
• Generates and evaluates solutions				
• Makes recommendations				
Interpersonal communication				
• Helps bringing out unspoken thoughts, issues and concerns				
• Explains specific veterinary medical information in easily understandable way				
• Practices attentive and active listening				
3. Advanced Competencies				
Leadership				
• Creates vision				
• Communicates vision and mission to team				
• Understands and uses team's capabilities				
Project Management				
• Gets together different work processes in a project				
• Controls, reviews and monitors progress				
• Controls quality and budget				
Adaptability				
• Be flexible during change				
• Thrives in changing work environment				
• Remains enthusiastic				
Change Management				
• Embraces change				
• Creates and supports flexibility				
• Presents realities of change				
Developing Self				
• Stays updated of latest research				
• Identifies emerging new requirements				
• Develops new skills				
Developing Subordinates				
• Identifies high potential employees				
• Ensures availability and time				
• Creates teams with complementary skill sets				
4. Technical Skills				
• Recognizes condition requiring surgeries				

Performance Appraisal for 2012 For Dr. Jane Bond Veterinary Surgeon	Excellent	Good	Average	Poor
• Demonstrates surgical skills and expertise				
• Demonstrates clinical skills and expertise				
• Monitors and evaluates high standards of medical care				
5. Personal Development				
• Proficiency in ultrasound examination through external training courses				
• Knowledge of major surgical methods				
• Knowledge of latest feline infectious diseases treatment approaches				
• Independent handling of night duties and emergencies				
Date:				
Appraiser (name and signature)				
Appraisee (name and signature)				

7.8. STAFF REWARDS

Staff rewards like salary increases or promotions depend on the quality of work, motivation, creativity and positive measurable impact of the staff on the veterinary practice. It should be given when the employee exceeds his or her expected work responsibilities and contributes to increased business profit, reputation and customer satisfaction. Promotions can be given following continued professional education, which adds value to the veterinary practice by acquiring new business fields that did not exist before. This can be in the form of additional qualifications like nutrition, behavior, dog grooming and dog training but also medical advancement like ophthalmology, dentistry, dermatology and new surgical techniques. Natural healing methods are very much blossoming now and are widely expected from customers. This opens a wide field of continued professional development thus resulting in promotions.

For small veterinary practices, online courses for professional education open the way to enhance employee's knowledge for a relatively fair amount of fees without losing valuable working time caused by employee's absenteeism. Although not all subjects can be learnt via long distance methods, it will help to support the gathering of theoretical background knowledge in a self-paced way. This can then be topped with a practical professional course as the reward for the employee that will be still feasible money-wise for even a small veterinary practice.

Monetary rewards like salary increases can be created in the form of bonus payments at the end of the year when certain clearly defined yearly targets have been met. It is useful to establish a set target of X % increase in annual profits compared to the previous year. A pre-defined bonus, e.g. of ½ or one monthly salary will be given if the set target has been reached the year's end, and the performance of the employee contributed to the achievement. This has the advantage that staff will be very motivated to reach the set target which will lead to a visible increase of their efforts, dedication, and work morale as well as client satisfaction.

The introduction of the "Employee of the Month/Quarter/Year" depending on the size of the veterinary practice is another reward tool that does not have a major monetary impact. The employee can be recognized by a small pecuniary amount or gift voucher. Moreover, the picture of the awarded employee can be hung in the reception area to make him/her visible to outside customers. This enhances pride, loyalty, commitment and motivation.

7.9. EMPLOYEE SATISFACTION SURVEY

Employee satisfaction surveys are an extremely powerful tool to assess the happiness, satisfaction and commitment of employees. They can be conducted on annual basis either in a formal or casual way. The formal way is a written questionnaire where employees are asked questions regarding their satisfaction with job conditions, salaries, workload and work conditions. Moreover, the survey includes questions regarding the trust in management, motivation and commitment to work and practice. The answers of these questionnaires provide valuable insight into the employees' thinking and feeling. Results can be used as basis for improvements in workflow, team work and attitude towards employees and among them. Another positive aspect is the fact that happy and satisfied team members are less likely to leave the veterinary practice any time soon.

Employee satisfaction surveys may contain a few questions but can also include several pages of questions. Short and concise questionnaires usually are sufficient to get a clear information what employees are thinking and feeling about their work in the veterinary practice.

Table 7.9. Sample Employee Satisfaction Survey

	Yes	No	Sometimes	Not sure
Do you feel valued?				
Do you feel that your work is appreciated?				
Do you feel that you contribute positively to the practice?				
Do you like your job?				
Do you feel overworked?				
Do you feel trained enough to do your job?				
Do you think that you require more training?				
Do you think that you should have more responsibilities?				
Are you treated fairly?				
Do you trust your superior?				
Do you trust the management?				
Do you feel proud of your work?				
Do you feel proud of the practice?				
Are you planning to leave the practice in the near future?				

7.10. CONCLUSION

Every organization and thus the veterinary practice depend on each individual team member. An excellent high-performance team has to be nurtured and cared for when expecting it to give 100% to its employer. This starts by deciding at what point of time to recruit new staff in order to be viable and profitable for the practice. Then it continues by selecting the right candidate for a job vacancy who fits into the existing team and complements it. Although easier said than done, the selections and recruitment process for a new employee is crucial for the future success of the veterinary practice. An unsuitable new staff can damage well functioning team structures and work processes and thus demolish the established work routine with subsequent negative impact on practice work, clients and profits. Once a suitable employee is found, a well-defined job description helps tremendously to clarify the type of work expected and to integrate the person into the practice team. Competencies or so-called soft skills are another important factor as no veterinary personnel lives from technical skills and knowledge alone in such a client-oriented profession. Loyalty, integrity, trust and client orientation are among the most important character traits of ideal employees. Staff needs to be motivated when we expect them to outperform themselves. This can be done in either monetary form or continued professional development. The latter is a critical factor in introducing new services as well as getting the competitive advantage towards other veterinary clinics. Usually, the advantages outweigh the disadvantages of training by far. Nowadays, either external training facilities as well as long distance online courses are available with a large variety of interesting and useful courses. Participation in training increases employee satisfaction and helps to retain excellent staff as pillars of the veterinary practice. Personal development plans identify knowledge gaps and tackle improvement measures with clearly defined action that are set with a timeline. They can be evaluated in performance appraisals whose results should flow into the employee reward scheme. Rewards are on one hand a great appreciation of hard work and outstanding performance and on the other hand, a marvelous motivator for further extraordinary and superior work. Annual employee satisfaction survey can prove to be an essential management tool to get a better understanding of what practice members think, need and want.

REFERENCES

[1]   Beech, N., Cairns, G., Livingstone, H., Lockyer, C. and Tsoukas, H. (2005). Managing people in organisations. Volume 2. The Graduate School of Business, University of Strathclyde, Glasgow, UK.

[2]   Brown, J.P. and Silverman,J.D.(1999). The current and future market for veterinarians and veterinary medical services in the United States. *JAVMA,* Vol. 215, No. 2, July 15. pp. 161-183.

[3]   Condra, M.E. and Howe, L. (2007). Increasing the impact of your healthcare organization's competency program. Healthstream. http://www.healthstream.com/ Libraries/whitePapers/Competency_Program.sflb.ashx (Accessed on August 10th, 2011).

[4]   CVE (2011). Centre for Veterinary Education. Long distance information. http://www.cve.edu.au/distanceeducation (Accessed on August 11th, 2011).

[5]   Eickemeyer (2011). Continuing Education: English Courses 2011 http://www.eickemeyerveterinary.com/education_english.php 47(Accessed on August 11th, 2011).

[6]   ESAVS (2011). European School for Advanced Veterinary Studies. Veterinary Courses and Workshops 2012. http://www.esavs.org/en/kategorie.php?k=47(Accessed on August 11th, 2011).

[7]   Gillespie, A. (1998). *Advanced Business Studies through diagrams.* Oxford University Press. UK.

[8]   Müller, M.G. and Abu Aabed, A. (2007). Guidelines for setting up a small and medium size enterprise. *MBA Thesis,* University of Strathclyde. Graduate School of Business. Glasgow, UK.

[9]   O'Shea, K. (2002).Staff Development Nursing Secrets. Philadelphia: Hanley & Belfus, Inc.

[10]   Ouwerkerk, M. and Schlegel, H. (1997). Erfolgreich Praxisfuehrung fuer den Tierarzt: Praxismanagament/ Praxismarketing. Hannover. Schluetersche GmbH.

[11]   Shilcock, M. and Stutchfield, G.(2005). *Veterinary practice management. A practical guide.* Reprinted, Saunders, Elsevier Ltd. Philadelphia.

[12]   Shilcock, M. and Stutchfield, G.(2008). *Veterinary practice management. A practical guide.* 2nd ed. Saunders, Elsevier Ltd. Philadelphia.

ACCOUNTING, MANAGEMENT ACCOUNTING AND BUDGETING

ABSTRACT

Accounting is definitely not one of the favored subjects for veterinarians and often delegated to the spouse of the owner or outsourced to local accounting boutiques. Yet, it is the most crucial areas for the survival of the veterinary practice.

This chapter provides detailed information about cash flows. It explains how they come together and what way exists of reading them. Moreover, this chapter explains the balance statements as well as the profit and loss statements as both are significant for controlling the business. Budgeting is another part of this accounting chapter.

8.1. INTRODUCTION

Accounting is for veterinarians often worse than performing the most difficult surgery. The long list of figures can frighten even the most capable veterinary surgeon. However, accounting is one of the most important works in veterinary practice. It is inevitable to get into financial accounting right from the start of setting up or purchasing the new veterinary practice.

Even for business planning, accounting figures are a must to develop a proper and well-founded business plan. This chapter aims at explaining the individual parts of the accounting sheets and to explain their validity and use in the veterinary practice context. This includes the cash flow statements explained step-by-step, its interpretation and importance for the business.

The balance sheet is explained in detail in an easily understandable way. The profit and loss or income statement is another important measure for veterinary practices. Inevitable for business, the budget and budgeting process is another part of this chapter. The accounting standard has been chosen according to the US Generally Accepted Accounting Principles (GAAP).

8.2. WHAT IS ACCOUNTING?

Accounting is defined as "collecting, analyzing and communicating financial information." [1, p.2]. This financial information is the basement for all financial decisions regarding development of introduction of new services or products, pricing of existing services or products, possible use of bank loan and operating capacity [1].

Through financial accounting, the consequences of decisions can be assessed [1] and better taken into consideration in a professional and future-oriented way. The step by step breakdown of accounting figures helps for a better understanding the usefulness of those numbers and to come to profound decision-making in the veterinary business.

However, it has to be made clear for which addressee and for which purpose the accounting figures are prepared as this varies among user groups as a variety of different accounting types exist such as bookkeeping, tax accounting and management accounting. It can be regarded as a kind of service as it provides financial data for a variety of users. Data used for financial accounting has to be reliable, relevant, comparable and easily understandable to be helpful for its users [1]. In addition, the method of data compilation must be consistent and in accordance with the local accounting regulations.

Accounting is differentiated into financial accounting and management accounting. This chapter contains information about management accounting. Financial accounting is explained in detail in the Chapter 9 "Finance, Financial Accounting and Financial Management" of this book. Whereas financial accounting serves for a variety of stakeholders, management accounting serves mainly the concerned manager and is intended for internal use in order to facilitate decision making. Therefore, the financial reports generated vary in terms of report types, time line, information quality, detail levels and degree of standardization [1].

While going through the individual part of accounting sheets, you will see that accounting is not so difficult and can be easily understood. In this chapter, the major financial accounting statements like cash flow statement, profit and loss statement and balance sheet will be explained in detail. All statements should be viewed together and not separate [1] in order to gain a complete overview of the financial situation of the veterinary practice.

Nowadays, excellent accounting software is available in the market that can be highly recommended. They can even replace an accountant in a small veterinary practice. Moreover, the costs for those software programs are affordable and provide the complete statements and report that are required for professional accounting. The only point to keep in mind is the fact that data entry has to be performed on a daily basis to get correct figures.

8.3. CASH FLOW

8.3.1. Cash Flow Statement

The cash flow statement states as per its name the movement of cash. Cash money is extremely important for the effective functioning of the veterinary practice and is therefore given highest importance as the main backbone of the business. It is used to e.g. to pay debts and to purchase items like medicines and inventories. Therefore, cash flow statements and charts provide extremely valuable information about the state of the business beyond information stated in profit and loss sheet or balance sheet. Analyzing cash flows provide a deeper understanding of where the business goes. The cash flow statement covers the flow of cash or wealth during a defined period like one day, one moth or one year. However, the cash flow statement should not be misunderstood as giving exclusive information about the health status of the business [1].

Cash can come from various sources such as operating activities, investing activities and financing activities. These three categories together add up to the net increase in cash over as period of time [1].

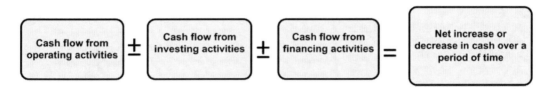

Figure 8.1. Cash flow statement layout [modified from 1].

Cash flow statements provide information for veterinary practice owners or manager if sufficient cash reserves are available for a potential expansion of the business. They are an important source of information for suppliers who would like to know if the veterinary practice has sufficient cash if they offer it to pay for supplies by credit. Employees might be interested in cash flow statements as they indicate if the practice can fund its operations and employees.

But from where does the cash flow come and where does it go? Cash comes from operating and financing activities and is then invested in investing activities [1]. Business events like repayment of loans or buying inventories have effects on the cash flow and profit. Those events differ very much with regard to their impact on profit and cash flow.

Table 8.1. Effects on cash flow and profit [1]

Events	Effect on profit	Effect on cash flow
Repayment of loan	None	Decrease
Buying a non-current asset for cash	None	Decrease
Making sale on credit	Increase	None
Buying inventories for cash	None	Decrease
Receiving cash from debtor	None	Increase
Depreciating a non-current asset	Decrease	None

How does the cash flow move over a period of time? What is the opening and closing balance on consecutive days? The example will illustrate the changes in the cash flow statement over a period of three days.

In our sample, the opening cash balance of the next day is the closing cash balance of the previous day which is 180 US $. If the income has not been deposited in the bank on the same day, the 180 US $ is then the closing cash balance at the end of day 1 and in the same time the opening cash balance of day 2.

Table 8.2. Sample cash flow statement for day 1 [modified from 1]

Cash flow statement for day 1	
	US $
Opening balance	100
+ cash from sales of pet accessories	200
	300
-cash paid to purchase the pet accessories	120
Closing cash balance	180
Income statement for day 1	
	US $
Sales revenue	180
- cost of pet accessories sold (3/4 of 120 US$)	90
Profit	90
Balance sheet at the end of day 1	
	US $
Cash of closing balance	180
Inventories of pet accessories sold (1/4 of 120 US$)	30
Total veterinary practice wealth	210

Table 8.3. Sample cash flow statement for day 2 [modified from 1]

Cash flow statement for day 2	
	US $
Opening balance	180
+ cash from sales of pet accessories	100
	280
-cash paid to purchase the pet accessories	40
Closing cash balance	240
Income statement for day 2	
	US $
Sales revenue	240
- cost of pet accessories sold (3/4 of 40 US$)	30
Profit	210
Balance sheet at the end of day 2	
	US $
Cash of closing balance	240
Inventories of pet accessories sold (1/4 of 40 US$)	10
Total veterinary practice wealth	250

In our sample, the opening cash balance of the third day is the closing cash balance of the second day which is 240 US $. If the income has not been deposited in the bank on the same day, the 240 US $ is, then the closing cash balance at the end of day 2 and in the same time the opening cash balance of day 3.

8.3.2. Cash Flow Chart

The protected cash flow can be shown in a chart that includes cash balance and net cash flow. Especially for smaller veterinary practices it should never be forgotten that cash is the most important thing to keep the business going. Just remember the old proverb "cash is king!", nothing can be truer than that. Following the detailed cash flow chart, a diagram of projected monthly cash flows can be developed, which clearly visualizes the net cash flow and cash balance. For every business plan that is either set up for opening a new veterinary practice or as forecasting tool, the pro forma cash flow for 3 years should be established.

Table 8.4. Sample cash flow statement for day 3 [modified from 1]

Cash flow statement for day 3	
	US $
Opening balance	240
+ cash from sales of pet accessories	160
	400
-cash paid to purchase the pet accessories	100
Closing cash balance	300
Income statement for day 3	
	US $
Sales revenue	300
- cost of pet accessories sold (3/4 of 100 US$)	75
Profit	225
Balance sheet at the end of day 3	
	US $
Cash of closing balance	300
Inventories of pet accessories sold (1/4 of 120 US$)	25
Total veterinary practice wealth	325

8.3.3. Analyzing Cash Flows

Now all cash flow data are broken down in a clearly understandable form. But what is the next step? How can the data be put together to complete the big picture of cash flows? This requires four main steps [4].

As the first step, the big picture has to be scanned and understood [4]. This works in the way that the veterinary practice is placed in the context in terms of age, size and other veterinary businesses. The annual report and other accounting reports of the veterinary practice are assessed [4] to determine the practice management has seen the year's progress. This shows if it has been a good year or even a record-breaking year in terms of revenue or net income [4]. On the other hand, there might have been difficult times [4] or even losses. The net income is the next record to look at. Here, it is interesting to review if the net income shows increases or losses over the past few years and if the income or loss is increasing or decreasing [4].

The second step in analyzing cash flows is to understand that the cash flow from operating activities is the cash flow engine of the practice [4]. When working effectively, the cash flow engine produces the cash flows to cover the cash needs of operations [4] in the veterinary practice. It is now essential to check if the cash flow from operating activities is greater than zero, and if it is increasing or decreasing [4]. For positive cash flows, the question arises whether they can cover important routine expenditures [4].

Table 8.5. Sample cash flow chart for 12 months

Month	Pre-start	1	2	3	4	5	6	7	8	9	10	11	12	Totals
Income														
Sales -cash														
Sales-credit														
Capital put in by owner														
Government start-up loan														
Bank loan														
A. Total Income														
Expenditure														
Materials -cash														
Materials-credit														
Rent and rates														
Electricity & heating														
Wages & salaries (net)														
Bank charges &interest														
Insurance														
Vehicle costs e.g. petrol														
Business travel														
Postage														
Stationary & printing														
Advertising														
Telephone calls														
Telephone line rental														
Internet connection														
Loan repayments														
Leasing charges														
Professional fees (for accountant)														
Capital expenditure - assets														
Personal drawings														
B. Total expenditure														
Net cash flow (A-B)														
Balance														
Closing balance														

Newly established veterinary practice are an exception to this rule as start-up businesses are often suffering from negative cash flows from operating activities. This is caused by high expenditure when setting up the new practice, and their cash flow engines are not yet up to full speed [4]. Lastly, the operating working capital accounts like inventories, receivables, and accounts payable should be examined as they usually increase in expanding companies [4].

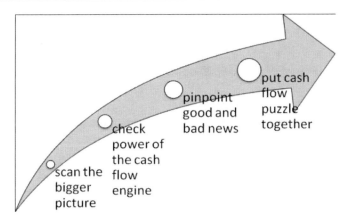

Figure 8.2. Analyzing cash flows.

As third step, good news and bad news are pinpointed [4]. To begin with, the cash flow from investing activities needs to be reviewed. One routine observation should be to examine whether the veterinary practice generates or uses its cash money for investing in assets. A healthy business invests continually to replace the assets that have become technologically outdated [4], old or damaged.

In veterinary practices this relates mainly to investments in more equipment, new or extended premises and land as well as other fixed assets. Now the entire investing cash flow needs to be reviewed. This helps to evaluate whether cash flows from financing belong to the "good news" or "bad news" categories [4]. One way is to compare loans, borrowing and payments on debt with each other across the years and evaluate if there are any trends. The other systematic way takes the route from activities in the stock accounts to discover news in this area [4].

Putting the puzzle pieces together is the final step [4]. It should not be believed that it is normal to find all examined cash flow movements either in positive or negative ways as this is very hard to find.

In contrast, a well-balanced evaluation is founded on the use of both, good news and bad news, that have been identified in each section of the cash flow statement [4]. In case of unclear, unusual or unknown items that may require further investigation or clarification, advice should be sought from a professional [4], e.g. certified public accountant.

8.4. BALANCE SHEET

The balance sheet "shows the financial position of an organisation at a particular moment in time" [3, p.37] and poses "a snapshot of the accounting records of assets, liabilities and capital of a business at a particular moment, most obviously the accounting year end." [7, p.51]. Moreover, the sources of finance for the practice like liabilities, either current or long-term, and capitals are a part of the balance sheet [1, 3]. This leads to the question what are assets, liabilities and capital?

8.4.1. Assets

Assets can be described as items that are possessed by the veterinary practice. They can be differentiated into tangible and intangible assets. Tangible assets being touchable assets of physical nature [1] include machinery and equipment, furniture and fixtures, vehicles, inventories or stock. In contrast, intangible assets do not possess physical nature and include e.g. patents, trademarks [1] and goodwill [9].

Another differentiation of assets is the grouping in current and fixed assets. Fixed assets are items that last for a longer period of time and at least more than 12 months. They usually include machinery and equipment, fixtures and furniture, vehicles and practice building [9]. Many fixed assets like vehicles, furniture and equipments lose their value from year to year. This process is called depreciation. Over a certain period of time, fixed assets will reach a value of zero when they are fully depreciated. This will be visible in the balance sheet where the cost of the fixed asset minus the depreciation is shown. Current assets include items that will be transformed into cash money within one year's time like stock items, cash, bank balances and debtors [9].

8.4.2. Liabilities

Liabilities are defined as claims of organizations, banks and individuals other than the owner against the business [1], e.g. bank loans or medicine supplies. They describe the amount of money that is owed by the veterinary practice to its creditors. Liabilities can be differentiated into current and long-term liabilities.

Current liabilities have the same time frame as current assets being the period of the next one year of the balance sheet date [1]. Until that time, the payment of the liability has to be paid. Current liabilities are mainly for trading purposes and cannot be deferred for more than 12 months after the balance sheet date [1]. This includes payments such as VAT, taxes, insurances, suppliers, laboratories, overdrafts and rents (accruals) [9]. It is useful to compare the current liabilities with the current assets as this is the cash inflow to meet the current liabilities [1].

In contrast, long-term liabilities are all liabilities that do not fall under the definition of current liabilities [1]. The time frame of the payment of long-term liabilities goes beyond one year. They contain usually larger sums of money for loans, mortgages and long-term finance for equipments and vehicles [9]. However, it should be reviewed to which extent the veterinary practice is financed by long-term liabilities compared to owner's capital. The more long-term liabilities exist, the higher the potential risk will be to meet those obligations in future [1].

8.4.3. Capital

Capital [9] or owner's claims [1] are another part of the balance sheet. The owner of the veterinary practice has invested his own money as stake in the veterinary practice which means that the practice owes him money. The distribution of capital depends on the legal form of the veterinary practice, e.g. sole ownership, joint partnership or limited company.

Table 8.6. Sample balance sheet for single ownership
[modified for veterinary practice from 1]

Happy Veterinary Practice (Bond DVM) Balance sheet as of 31st December 2011		
	000 US $	000 US $
Fixed assets		
Buildings and premises		111
Fixtures, furniture and fittings		42
Motor vehicles		22
		175
Current assets		
Inventories (stock)	18	
Trade receivables (debtors)	13	
Cash at bank	2	
Prepayments	1	
	34	
Less current liabilities		
Trade payables (creditors)	28	
Overdraft	4	
Accruals	1	
	(33)	
Total assets less current liabilities		176
Long-term liabilities		
Bank loan		(65)
Total net assets		101
Capital		
Opening balance		80
Add profit		23
		103
Less drawings		2
		101

According to this legal framework, the capital will be broken down further in the balance sheet. For single ownership and joint ownership, the capital is composed of two parts, the capital account and the current account [9]. The capital account is the long-term investment in the veterinary practice whereas the current account represents the profit shares. In case of limited companies, the investment of the owners is reflected as share capital in the balance sheet [9].

Goodwill is a special intangible asset. It is not shown normally in the balance sheet, but it comes into effect at the time of sale of the veterinary practice. Goodwill includes the customer relations, reputation of the practice and staff skill and quality of veterinary services. Goodwill cannot be measured or verified, and therefore, it has to be agreed on its value [1] when the veterinary practice will be sold. As it then does have a fixed price, goodwill finds its way into the balance sheet as a fixed asset by the practice that bought it [1].

Table 8.7. Sample balance sheet for joint ownership of two partners at time of sale [modified for veterinary practice from 1]

Happy Veterinary Practice(Bond and Smith DVMs)Balance sheet as of 31st December 2011		
	000 US $	000 US $
Fixed assets		
Buildings and premises		100
Goodwill		11
Fixtures, furniture and fittings		42
Motor vehicles		22
		175
Current assets		
Inventories (stock)	18	
Trade receivables (debtors)	13	
Cash at bank	2	
Prepayments	1	
	34	
Less current liabilities		
Trade payables (creditors)	28	
Overdraft	4	
Accruals	1	
	(33)	
Total assets less current liabilities		176
Long-term liabilities		
Bank loan		(65)
Total net assets		101
Partner's Capital		
Opening balance Bond		50
Opening balance Hyde		30
Add profit		23
		103
Less drawings		2
		101

8.5. PROFIT AND LOSS STATEMENT OR INCOME STATEMENT

The income statement or profit and loss statement has the function "to measure and report how much profit (wealth) the business has generated over a period" [1, p.62]. It gives information when a profit will be reached [8]. Both, expenses and revenue need to be identified, expenses being defined as the "inflow of economic benefits arising from the ordinary activities of a business" [1, p.62] which might include e.g. value of product sales and services income [1, 3].

Table 8.8. Profit and Loss Statement [modified for veterinary practice from 1]

Happy Veterinary Practice Bond DVM Income statement for the year ended 31 December 2011	US $	US $
Turnover		480,000
Less Cost of sales		(152,000)
Gross profit		328,000
Less		
Salaries and wages	145,000	
Rent and rates	35,000	
Heat and light	4,200	
Telephone	2,800	
Postage, stationary	2,500	
Insurance	2,000	
Motor vehicles	6,500	
Loan interest	4,000	
CPD	1,000	
Depreciation	1,000	
		(204,000)

8.6. BUDGETING

8.6.1. General Information

The budget preparation is important for future plans. Budgets are described as "a detailed statement of financial results expected for a given future period" [5, p.343] and are helpful in the co-ordination of various business parts, encouraging better performance among managers, helping in identifying short-term problems and serving as authorization systems [1]. In order to control the financial activities of a small business, budgets form the basis of the budgetary control which evaluates the development of the finances according to the set plans [5].

Budgeting is essential to control the financial performance of the veterinary practice. Although budgeting might be a field that is sometimes not well-liked and fully understood especially by inexperienced veterinarians, it will provide vital information about the financial status of the practice [6]. Typically, budgets are divided into long-term budget plans of up to five years and short-term budget for 12 months [1]. A contingency of up to 10% can be helpful to cover unexpected and not budgeted expenses like replacement of damaged equipment.

The budget contains different kinds of budgets like the operating and financial budget which are summarized in the master budget [2].

The financial budget includes capital budget and cash budget that gets consolidated in the budgeted balance sheet. Sales budget and costs budget lead to a budgeted profit and loss statement that provides information about financial results in the future. The budgeted profit and loss flows also in the budgeted balance sheet [2].

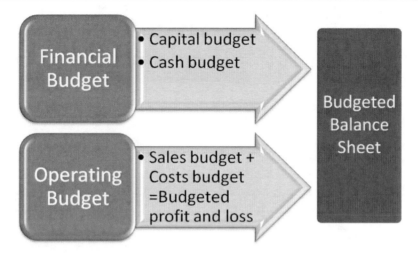

Figure 8.3. Overview of budget composition [modified from 2, p.167].

8.6.2. Cash Budget

The cash budget is one of the most important budgets that needs to be prepared. Usually, it is prepared before the other budgets are done because it is regarded as the key budget. The cash budget shows the economic business aspects more than any other budget [1]. Different budget styles and time periods do exist and depend largely on the veterinary practice itself as budgets are for internal use. Cash budgets are normally prepared according to months. It is divided into received cash and payment of cash. Cash surplus is defined as total cash receipts over payments or of payments over receipts and calculated for each single month [1]. Cash surplus and the opening cash balance of the previous month equals the closing cash balance which is the running cash [1]. The cash budget is based on the figures of the income statement and cash movements during a given period of time. This can be seen in detail explained in an example.

8.6.3. Other Budgets

Apart from the cash budget, other budget are the

- Capital budget
- Operational budget
- Manpower budget
- Trade Receivables budgets
- Trade Payables budgets
- Inventories budgets

The capital budget includes all capital equipments and machinery, vehicles, buildings, computer hardware and software as well as any other capital item. The operational budget covers operational expenses and running costs of the veterinary practice. The manpower budget contains any staff-related costs like salaries, insurances and pensions as well as the new recruitments.

Table 8.9. Sample cash budget for 6 months
[modified for veterinary practice from 1]

The Happy Veterinary Practice has the following budgeted income statement for 6 months:						
Income statement (January to June)						
Months	Jan	Feb	Mar	Apr	May	June
	US $ 000	US $ 000	US $ 000	US $ 000	US $ 000	US $ 000
Revenue from						
Treatment	40	45	45	52	55	48
Medicines+ accessories sales	20	22	25	18	23	25
Total revenue	60	67	70	60	78	73
Cost of goods sold	10	11	12	9	11	13
Salaries	35	35	35	35	35	35
Electricity	5	5	5	5	5	5
Depreciation	2	2	2	2	2	2
Other overheads	2	2	2	2	2	2
Total expenses	54	55	56	53	55	57
Net profit	6	12	14	7	23	16
Happy Veterinary Practice offers one month credit for its clients so that the cash from January is received in February. Therefore the receivables in the cash budget are lagging one month behind. In December, the revenue was US $ 80,000. Electricity is paid quarterly in March and June. A new vehicle for the practice has to be bought for US $ 18,000 in February and the old one will be taken into commission for US$ 2,000. The cash balance at start of January was US $14,000. The cash balance of each month is the previous month's balance plus cash surplus. The cash budget looks now as follows:						
Cash Budget (January to June)						
Months	Jan	Feb	Mar	Apr	May	June
	US $ 000	US $ 000	US $ 000	US $ 000	US $ 000	US $ 000
Receipts						
Receivables	80	60	67	70	60	78
Payments						
Payables	10	10	11	12	9	11
Salaries	35	35	35	35	35	35
Electricity	-	-	15	-	-	15
Other overheads	2	2	2	2	2	2
Vehicle purchase		16				
Total payments	47	63	63	49	46	63
Cash surplus	33	(3)	4	21	14	15
Opening balance	12	9	13	24	38	53
Closing balance	45	6	17	25	52	68

Table 8.10. Sample budget sheet for 12 months [modified for veterinary practice from 1]

	Happy Veterinary Practice Budget 2012												
	Quarter 1			Quarter 2			Quarter 3			Quarter 4			
Months	1	2	3	4	5	6	7	8	9	10	11	12	Total
Description													
Capital Expenditure													
Buildings													
Vehicles													
Equipment													
Practice Fixtures and Furniture													
Computers & printers													
Computer softwares													
Total Capital Cost													
Operational Expenditure													
Rent and rates													
Electricity & heating													
Water													
Bank charges &interest													
Insurances													
Vehicle costs e.g. petrol													
Business travel													
Courier & Postage													
Stationary													
Publications & printing													
Advertising													
Telephone calls													
Telephone line rental													
Internet connection													
Loan repayments													
Leasing charges													
Professional fees (for accountant)													
Practice Maintenance													
Books & Journals													
Consumables													
Laboratory Consumables													
Animal Food													
Tools													
Construction & modification													
Maintenance													
Total Operating Cost													
Manpower Cost													
Salaries													
Insurances													
Health insurances													

Happy Veterinary Practice Budget 2012												
	Quarter 1			Quarter 2			Quarter 3			Quarter 4			
Months	1	2	3	4	5	6	7	8	9	10	11	12	Total
Health insurances													
Overtime													
Pension													
Recruitment													
Training charges													
Total Manpower Cost													
Grand Total													

Table 8.11. Sample trade receivables budget, trade payables budget and inventories budget for 6 months [modified for veterinary practice from 1]

Trade Receivables Budget (January to June)						
Months	Jan	Feb	Mar	Apr	May	June
	US $ 000	US $ 000	US $ 000	US $ 000	US $ 000	US $ 000
Opening balance	80	60	67	70	60	78
Add sales revenue	60	67	70	60	78	73
	140	127	137	130	138	151
Less cash receipts	80	60	67	70	60	78
Closing balance	60	67	70	60	78	73
Trade Payables Budget (January to June)						
Months	Jan	Feb	Mar	Apr	May	June
	US $ 000	US $ 000	US $ 000	US $ 000	US $ 000	US $ 000
Opening balance	10	10	11	12	9	11
Add purchases	10	11	12	9	11	10
	20	21	23	21	20	21
Less cash payment	10	10	11	12	9	11
Closing balance	30	31	34	33	29	32
Inventories Budget (January to June)						
Months	Jan	Feb	Mar	Apr	May	June
	US $ 000	US $ 000	US $ 000	US $ 000	US $ 000	US $ 000
Opening balance	12	12	12	8	8	8
Add purchases	10	11	12	9	11	10
	12	23	24	17	19	18
Less inventories used	10	11	12	9	11	13
Closing balance	22	34	36	26	30	31

The trade receivables' budget contains the planned amount from credit sales at the beginning and end of each month as well as the planned monthly sales revenue and planned total cash receipts from receivables [1].

The trade payables budget is the planned amount owed to suppliers by the veterinary practice at beginning and end of each month, the planned monthly purchases and planned total cash payments to payables [1].

The inventories' budget includes the planned amount of inventories that the practice holds at the beginning and end of each month, the planned total monthly purchases and planned total inventory's usage per month [1].

All three budgets are interconnected to each other as well as to the cash budget that was described in detail above in this chapter. Therefore, identical rows of figures can be seen as follows:

- Purchase figures rows: in payables budget and inventories budget [1]
- Cash payment figures rows: in payables budget and cash budget [1]
- Cash receipts figures rows: in receivables budget and cash budget [1]
- Cost of goods sold figure in budgeted income statement is identical with less inventories used figure in inventories budget

8.7. CONCLUSION

Accounting is one of the most important parts in veterinary business, although veterinarians find it usually very difficult to understand. Excellent accounting software is available and provide tremendous support with a full range of reports and statements. In every practice, major importance is placed on the cash flows as they are vital for its liquidity. However, it is not just significant to have cash flows but also to read them correctly.

The balance sheet is a main statement as it includes the practice's assets and capital as well as liabilities. The profit and loss statement measures the profit that the veterinary practice has generated over a certain time. With regard to budgeting, the budget forms another essential part of accounting as it gives a forecast of the required money in the coming years and its allocation to various cost centers.

REFERENCES

[1]   Atrill, P. and McLaney, E. (2006). Accounting and finance for non-specialists. 5th ed. *Financial Times*. Prentice Hall. Essex. UK.

[2]   Ciancanelli, P., Dunn, J., Koch, B. and M. Stewart (2006). Financial and management accounting. 4th ed. Glasgow: *The Graduate School of Business University of Strathclyde.*

[3]   Gillespie, A. (1998). Advanced Business Studies through diagrams. Oxford University Press. UK.

[4]   Hertenstein, J.H. and McKinnon, S. (1997). *Solving the puzzle of the cash flow statement. Reprinted from Business Horizons.* January/February. pp. 69-76. http://isites.harvard.edu/fs/docs/icb.topic498331.files/Puzzle%20of%20the%20Cash%20Flow%20Stmt.pdf (Accessed on August 12th, 2012).

[5]   Megginson, W.L., Byrd, M.J. and Megginson, L.C. (2000). *Small business management: An entrepreneur's guidebook.* 3rd ed. McGraw-Hill. Boston, Madrid, Toronto.

[6] Müller, M.G. and Abu Aabed, A. (2007). Guidelines for setting up a small and medium size enterprise. *MBA Thesis, University of Strathclyde.* Graduate School of Business. Glasgow, UK.

[7] Nobes, C. (1995). *The economist books: Pocket accounting.Penguin Group.* Hamondsworth, Middlesex, England.

[8] Ryan, J.D. and Hiduke, G.P. (2006). *Small business: an entrepreneur's business plan.* 7th ed. Thompson Soth-Western. Ohio.

[9] Shilcock, M. and Stutchfield, G.(2008). *Veterinary practice management. A practical guide.* 2nd ed. Saunders, Elsevier Ltd. Philadelphia.

Chapter 9

FINANCE, FINANCIAL ACCOUNTING AND FINANCIAL MANAGEMENT

ABSTRACT

Financial figures and ratios are inevitable features of veterinary practice management. It is imperative for every practice owner or manager to understand fully the different ratios and their use. They are divided in profitability measures, efficiency ratios and liquidity rations. Moreover, the long-term debts and financial gearing are important for long-term planning of the practice. The success of the veterinary practice depends on proper understanding of figures as they are required to get an overview of the veterinary business' performance. Only by understanding ratios, corrective actions can be taken to increase profitability and enhance efficiency and liquidity being the key performance parameters of every veterinary practice. This will lead to the successful financial management of the veterinary practice. This chapter explains in detail the various ratios and parameters that are required to control the financial performance of veterinary practices.

9.1. INTRODUCTION

Often veterinary practitioners are overwhelmed by the huge amount of numbers in financial accounting and finance management. However, a structured approach towards financial data helps to find the way through the number jungle. Using financial ratios clarifies the finance position of the veterinary practice. It is inevitable to understand financial ratios in order to be able to define the business strategy and ways to enhance profitability, efficiency and liquidity.

Only too often veterinary practitioners and practice owners are intimidated by the sheer amount of figures that seem to be like a jungle without light. Even so, by going step by step, light starts to shed into the jungle and a clear picture of the financial situation of the practice arises. Understanding the basics in financial management helps to control the financial performance of veterinary practices and to see when something goes in the wrong direction. It is by far not enough just to be an excellent veterinary professional, financial knowledge is the key to successful practice management to guide the practice through good and bad times.

9.2. WHAT IS FINANCE?

Finance is defined as being "concerned with the ways in which funds for a business are raised and invested" [1, p.2]. It provides a help for better decision making, especially with regard to investment of funds in e.g. machinery and equipments, inventories and premises with the aim to increase the wealth of the investor [1], said a veterinary practice. It identifies the costs, benefits and risk of an investment as well as return on investment [1], all inevitable components to grow the veterinary business in as a sustainable way. Financial data is based on the accounting figures of the veterinary practice.

9.3. PROFIT PLANNING

9.3.1. Introduction to Profit Planning

Financial planning needs to reach a profitability line. Profit planning being "a series of prescribed steps to be taken to ensure that a profit will be made" can help in this endeavor [6, p.322]. These steps include the determination of the amount of profit and its achievability, setting up of a proper accounting system for the veterinary practice with interpretation of the financial figures and last, but not least the evaluation of the practice's financial position [6]. The profit is actually "the difference between revenues earned and expenses incurred" [6, p.329], which means the "excess of the revenues over the expenses of the period" [8,p.139]. Profit planning can be performed from the operational plan of a given future period of time.

If the outcome of this profit analysis does not match the expectations, the veterinary practitioner or practice manager has to readjust his profit planning. One way is to find other alternatives, which may help in boosting profits are new services or entirely different sources of income. Furthermore, it is important to evaluate the relation between the expenses and changes in the volume of services and product sale [6]. Other ways of increasing the profit are reduced planned expenses through better control systems, increased productivity of staff and machines as well as a reduction of variable costs and increased sale prices [6].

What are the steps for profit planning? First of all, the veterinary practice operations have to be evaluated. This includes the comparison of the actual revenue and costs with the projected income statement.

The income statement is explained in detail in Chapter 8 "Accounting, Management Accounting and Budgeting" in this book. Such a comparison leads to the detection of unsatisfactory performance to take corrective actions. As the second step the needs and requirements for additional resources have to be looked at which may include employing fresh staff or acquiring new practice premises. The third step in profit planning is the clear understanding and planning of required purchases like inventories.

The volume of sold inventories has to be reviewed before deciding on how many new items have to be purchased. Sometimes purchase of discounted bulk might add considerably to the profit of the veterinary practice. However, purchase of not used bulk quantities might destroy the planned profit. The optional fourth step is the use of external funds to put the practice on safe feet in times of crisis.

9.3.2. Advantages and Limitations of Profit Planning

The advantages of profit planning are manifold. First of all, it is a financial planning tool that provides information of required investment in inventory, personnel or premises facilities as well as additional capital. Furthermore, it helps to evaluate the performance of the veterinary practice and to compare if the planned and actual profit matches or not. Profit plans help to control unrealized excessive costs and spending. Potential problems and threats to the veterinary business can be detected early, and their extent can be evaluated and corrective actions taken. Profit planning can point at potential future opportunities that can help the practice to get more income and profit. This helps to plan ahead actively in the future and not just to wait until everything is passed by. Profit planning can be a useful tool when looking for a bank loan as it shows the bank the well-thought approach and future profits of the entity and encourages lending.

Limitations of profit planning exist as all profit plans are not based on actual data but on estimated figures. Therefore, the possibility arises that these forecasts may change due to unexpected circumstances. Especially in economically rough times, profit planning is influenced by a large variety of external factors and may not lead to the expected results. Currency instabilities and increased taxes may lead to price increases of items that were not expected. In such cases, profit plans need to be revised and adjusted to the actual situation and then planned new again. The word "plan" entails that a revision of it has to be done according to the circumstances. However, a well-though and realistic yearly profit plan can aid to better control for the veterinary business and its budgetary expenses.

Another vital point for the profit planning and survival and success of a business is the cash flow. Cash flow can be improved by relatively easy ways like increased cash sales of products and services. Additionally, early payments can be pushed with small incentives, overdrafts and business credit cards can be used, and many suppliers offer special trade credits [5] with extended payment periods. The cash flow is described in detail in Chapter 8 "Accounting, Management Accounting and Budgeting" in this book.

9.4. BREAK-EVEN ANALYSIS

The break-even analysis helps in projecting the point of time and required volume of sales of product or services when the new business will start to make money. The break-even point is defined as "that volume of sales where total revenue and expenses are equal, so there is neither profit or loss" [6, p.336]. Therefore, the calculation of the break-even point requires estimates of variable and fixed costs [1].

The definition of the break-even point is as follows [1]:

$$\text{Break - even point} = \frac{\text{Total fixed costs (TFC)}}{\text{Sales revenue per unit (SPU) - variable costs per unit (VCU)}}$$

In an example we assume that the monthly fixed costs of the newly opened veterinary practice are US $ 20,000. The average per unit revenue, for example consultation, is US $ 80 and the cost of it is US $ 20. The break-even calculation goes as follows:

$$\text{Break - even point} = \frac{20,000 \text{ US \$}}{(80 - 20) \text{ US \$}} = \frac{20,000 \text{ US \$}}{60 \text{ US \$}} = 333,33 \text{ units}$$

This means that the veterinary practice has to perform 333 units or consultations in this example per month in order to break even. The revenue of 333 units multiplied by US $ 80 per unit is US $ 26,667 monthly. Profit will be made when the number of 333 consultations is crossed or the revenue of the consultation is increased. The break-even point in US $ is calculated by multiplication of the break- even point in units by Sales revenue per unit.

Break-even point (in US $) = Break-even point (units) x Sales revenue per unit

In a Microsoft Excel chart, the break-even chart will then look as follows:

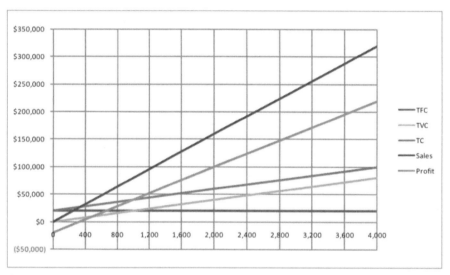

Break-Even Point (units) =333　　　　　**Break-Even Point ($'s) =$26,667**

Total Fixed CostsTFC =$20,000　　　　　Formulas:

Variable Cost per UnitVCU =$20.00　　　　BEP (units) = TFC/(SPU-VCU)

Sales Price per UnitSPU =$80.00　　　　BEP ($'s) = BEP (units) * SPU

Figure 9.1. Break-even chart.

9.5. FINANCIAL RATIOS

Although many different financial ratios do exist, only a few are really necessary to understand and control the small business. One of the most important profitability measures is the return on capital employed (ROCE) which is expressed in percentages [1]. Other important and relevant ratios are explained in detail in this chapter.

9.5.1. Profitability Ratio

9.5.1.1. Return On Capital Employed (ROCE) and Return on Equity (ROE)

Being regarded as "the most important profitability ratio" [3, p.84], the Return on Capital Employed or ROCE provides information about the amount of invested capital into a business and its generated returns [3]. This percentage ratio is derived from the net profit before interest and taxation [1] and covers the whole company's profitability [7]. However, the ratio can assess the individual parts of a business as well [3]. It reflects the efficiency of the investment to get revenue out of this investment [7, 10, 13]. The definition of ROCE is as follows [3, p.84].

$$ROCE = \frac{Net\ Profit\ before\ interest\ and\ tax}{Share\ capital + reserves + long\ term\ debt} \times 100$$

Another profitability measure is the Return on Shareholders' Funds (ROSF) or Return on Equity (ROE) stating the return on the investment by the shareholders. The ROSF/ROE can be kept by the company instead as being paid as dividends [3]. ROSF/ROE is defined as [3, p.84]:

$$ROSF/ROE = \frac{Profit\ after\ tax}{Share\ capital + reserves} \times 100$$

Both, ROCE and ROE are calculated from the balance sheet. However, the balance sheet is just a picture of the business at a fixed point of time and might not represent the real financial situation of the business throughout the year. This requires further performance measures at different times of the year [1]. Moreover, ROCE does not take hidden taxes into consideration [10].

Another general problem of ROCE is that it has many different definitions [3, 13], which makes it inevitable to keep the figures consistent [3]. One major issue with ROCE is the fact that this ratio is a measurement of the return against the book value of assets in the business. This creates problems with the depreciation because the depreciated assets lead to higher ROCE, although the cash flow is not affected [7]. This might give a wrong impression about older businesses with more depreciated assets and thus higher ROCE, although it is possible that some newer businesses might be better [7, 13].

Another problem of ROCE is that the book value of assets is not affected by inflation. However, inflation has a high impact on cash flow with increased revenues through inflation whereas ROCE stays unaffected [7, 13].

A further limitation of ROCE is the fact that goodwill, brand names [1], patents as well as copyrights [4] forming a considerable asset value are not accounted in the balance sheet. Therefore, ROCE does not consider those intangible assets [1]. Another issue of ROCE is the fact that some companies update the values of assets in the balance sheet regularly which leads to an increased ROCE [7]. As other businesses might not do the same, the comparison of those businesses might give a wrong conclusion [3].

Furthermore, a large practice with higher profit might have a lower ROCE compared to a small practice with lower profit, which requires a thorough look at the real business situation examined [1]. Moreover, the ROSF percentage does not give information about the amount of company's debts or shareholders' funds [7]. A high ratio of a company that has no debts might lead to possible wrong result interpretations [3, 7].

9.5.1.2. Net and Gross Profit Margin

The net and gross profit margins are both expressed in percentages. They provide information about the profit of the veterinary practice as a percentage of the sales revenue [1] or turnover [11]. The net profit margin states the net profit for a certain period to the turnover or sales revenue during the same period and is calculated as follows [1, 11]:

$$\text{Net profit margin} = \frac{\text{Net profit before interest and taxation}}{\text{Turnover (sales revenue)}} \times 100$$

The net profit margin ratio is often considered as the "most appropriate measure of operational performance" [1, p.177]. It is especially useful to compare the profitability development of the same veterinary practice over several years. However, it is not the best ratio to be used to compare the veterinary practice to other veterinary practices [11].

The gross profit margin ratio states the relation of the gross profit to the turnover or sales revenue in the same period of time and reflects differences between cost of sales and sales revenue. It is regarded as a profitability measure in purchasing and selling stock [1] like medicines or pet food before taking into account any other expenses [1]. It is highly important to understand the nature of the veterinary practice as this reflects in this ratio. A veterinary practice with a higher portion of laboratory costs or pet food sales will have a relatively lower gross profit margin due to the higher cost of sales [11]. The gross profit margin is defined as [1]:

$$\text{Gross profit margin} = \frac{\text{Gross profit}}{\text{Turnover (sales revenue)}} \times 100$$

9.5.2. Efficiency Ratios

Efficiency ratios are very important to assess the management of business resources. They include the average inventories (stock) turnover period, average settlement period for receivables, average settlement period for payables, sales revenue to capital employed and sales revenue per employee.

Average Inventories (Stock) Turnover Period

Inventories or stock are a major investment for the veterinary practice and pose a large amount of money that is fixed and cannot be used for anything else. Therefore, a quick turnaround of stock items is desirable and a period of 30 days should be attempted [1, 11]. The calculation for average inventories is done by taking the average of the opening and closing stock for the time period of one year [1]. In seasonal veterinary practices like large animal practices, the monthly average inventories can be taken to get more accurate figures.

The average inventories' turnover period gives the information about the time inventories are held. The ratio is calculated as follows [1]:

$$\text{Average inventories turnover period} = \frac{\text{Average inventories (stock) held}}{\text{Cost of sales}} \times 365$$

Average Settlement Period for Receivables

The average settlement period for receivables is a calculation about the time that it takes creditors to pay their payments that the veterinary practice has to receive from them. This is an important ratio as it determines the amount of cash flows [1] into the practice. Therefore, shorter receivables settlement periods are desirable as otherwise outstanding money is tied up for a too long time thus negatively impacting the cash flow of the practice. It should not be forgotten that few large customers with long payment delays can lead to massive extensions of days in this ratio.

The ratio is calculated as follows [1]:

$$\text{Average settlement period for receivables} = \frac{\text{Trade receivables}}{\text{Credit sales revenue}} \times 365$$

Average Settlement Period for Payables

Another valuable ratio is the average settlement period for payables. This ratio is the measurement of how long the veterinary practice takes to pay its outstanding amounts. Some practices regard the payment of outstanding settlements as a kind of free finance for their business and try to extend the average settlement period. However, one should consider that this might lead to problems with suppliers and the loss of good reputation of the veterinary practice with negative effects for practice-supplier relations. This ratio is as follows [1]:

$$\text{Average settlement period for payables} = \frac{\text{Trade payables}}{\text{Credit purchases}} \times 365$$

Sales Revenue to Capital Employed

The ratio of sales revenue to capital employed or asset turnover provides valuable information of the effective use of the practice's assets in order to generate turnover or sales revenues. In case of productive use of assets and therefore higher revenue generation, the ratio will be higher. The ratio is defined as follows [1]:

$$\text{Sales revenue to capital employed} = \frac{\text{Sales revenue}}{\text{Share capital} + \text{reserves} + \text{non-current liabilities}}$$

Sales Revenue Per Employee

The sales revenue per employee ratio measures the productivity of staff in relation to the sales revenue or turnover. A high ratio is definitely desired by practice owners and managers. The ratio is as follows [1]:

$$\text{Sales revenue per employee} = \frac{\text{Turnover (Sales revenue)}}{\text{Number of employees}}$$

However, the ratio cannot determine between the productivity of individual staff as it calculated only the overall productivity of all staff employed in the veterinary practice.

9.5.3. Liquidity Ratios

Another very important ratio is the liquidity ratio which gives information about the short-term financial obligation. The liquidity ratio is defined in two ratios, the current ratio and the acid test ratio [1].

Current Ratio

The current ratio provides information about the liquidity by comparing cash and assets that will be soon turned into cash with the current liabilities [1].

$$\text{Current ratio} = \frac{\text{Current assets}}{\text{Current liabilities}}$$

It helps the veterinary practice to get an indication about its liquidity status. The liquidity will be rated higher if the current ratio is higher. The ratio should be 1.5:1 [11] or up to 2:1 [1] as then the liquid assets are one and a half or twice the amount of the liabilities. This test provides information about the extensive use of overdraft facilities instead of use of long-term bank loans [11].

Acid Test

As inventories are often dead money for especially small businesses and cannot easily be immediately converted into cash, the acid tests' ratio takes this factor into consideration [1]. It is usually used as a variation of the current ratio excluding inventories and is defined as [1]:

$$\text{Acid test} = \frac{\text{Current assets (excluding inventories)}}{\text{Current liabilities}}$$

The acid test is regarded as a more stringent test than the current ratio [1, 11]. Its minimum level should be 1:1 or 1.0 times. This is the case when current assets excluding inventories equal current liabilities [1]. Nevertheless, fluctuations arising during the year have to be taken into consideration [11]. However, in reality, a lower ratio can be found without causing excessive cash-flow problems [1].

9.5.4. Financial Gearing

A measure for long-term planning is gearing. Gearing takes place when the owner of the practice cannot pay for the practice by his own finances and needs to borrow money, e.g. through bank loans. The level of gearing is highly important as it is closely linked with risk assessments. The higher the borrowing, the higher the risk of becoming insolvent in the future due to high interest rates and capital repayments [1]. Gearing is assessed in two ratios, the gearing ratio and interest cover ratio.

Gearing Ratio
The gearing ratio provides information about the borrowing to the long-term capital structure [1] of the veterinary practice. It is defined as [1]:

$$\text{Gearing ratio} = \frac{\text{Long-term liabilities}}{\text{Share capital + reserves + long-term liabilities}} \times 100$$

Interest Cover Ratio
The interest payable has to be covered by the amount of profit available. This is expressed in the interest cover ratio which is calculated as follows [1]:

$$\text{Interest cover ratio} = \frac{\text{Profit before interest and taxation}}{\text{Interest payable}}$$

9.5.5. Business Ratios

Ratios make sense when they are looked at in a common context. It does not really help to evaluate only one ration and neglect the others. The analysis of ratios compared two related figures that are usually coming from the same financial statement. They aid in understanding what the financial statements indicate. In order to have comparable data or benchmark ratios, performance of similar businesses and planned performance can be used from past periods. Financial statements can help in interpreting financial ratios or provide further data that are not given by ratios [1].

However, it should be clear that rations can only be as good as the financial statements they come from. Some ratios might be misleading as the balance sheet they come from provide solely a momentary picture of the business [1]. Another difficulty might be to get benchmark data from the veterinary industry.

After having the individual ratios, all ratios are put together to provide a clear picture of the veterinary practice's business state.

Table 9.1. Ratio analysis

Happy Veterinary Practice Bond DVM Ratio Analysis			
Ratio	Definition	Applied to veterinary practice	Results
Profitability Ratios			
ROCE	$\dfrac{\text{Net Profit before interest +tax}}{\text{(Share capital + reserves + long term debt)}} \times 100$		
ROSF/ROE	$\dfrac{\text{Profit after tax}}{\text{Share capital + reserves}} \times 100$		
Net profit margin	$\dfrac{\text{Net profit before interest+taxation}}{\text{Turnover (sales revenue)}} \times 100$		
Gross profit margin	$\dfrac{\text{Gross profit}}{\text{Turnover (sales revenue)}} \times 100$		
Efficiency ratios			
Average inventories turnover period	$\dfrac{\text{Average inventories (stock) held}}{\text{Cost of sales}} \times 365$		
Average settlement period for receivables	$\dfrac{\text{Trade receivables}}{\text{Credit sales revenue}} \times 365$		
Average settlement period for payables	$\dfrac{\text{Trade payables}}{\text{Credit purchases}} \times 365$		
Sales revenue to capital employed	$\dfrac{\text{Sales revenue}}{\text{Share capital+reserves+non-current Liabilities}}$		
Sales revenue per employee	$\dfrac{\text{Turnover (sales revenue)}}{\text{Number of employees}}$		
Liquidity ratios			
Current ratio	$\dfrac{\text{Current assets}}{\text{Current liabilities}}$		
Acid test	$\dfrac{\text{Current assets (excl. inventories)}}{\text{Current liabilities}}$		
Financial Gearing			
Gearing ratio	$\dfrac{\text{Long-term liabilities}}{\text{(Share capital+reserves+long-term Liabilities)}} \times 100$		
Interest cover ratio	$\dfrac{\text{Profit before interest+taxation}}{\text{Interest payable}}$		

9.6. PRICING

One of the major guidelines for successful businesses is not to price too low in the beginning as it is very difficult to raise the prices afterwards. Moreover, all costs need to be covered in order not to make a loss. However, pricing is not something static, but needs to be revised according to the inflation rate, economic situation or competition [12].

There are different pricing methods for products such as cost-plus pricing, demand pricing, competitive pricing and mark-up pricing [12]. Cost-plus pricing covers the cost of the product plus the overhead and the profit. Overhead includes fixed expenses like rent, salaries, liabilities, insurances as well as variable expenses such as phone bills, stationary, printing costs, etc. Another used pricing method is mark-up pricing, which is expressed as the percentage of the cost [12] that is added to the cost price to give the selling price. Therefore, the mark-up pricing is the profit in percentages of the cost. In contrast, the margin is the percentage of the selling price that serves as profit [11].

"veterinary service prices have not risen as fast as the general consumer prices since at least 1972... it is likely that supply pressure has led to excess capacity and subsequent downward price pressure..." [2, p.165]. This poses a major problem for veterinarians as there is a strong correlation between the development of the veterinary market and the price structure of services. Many individual veterinarians are forced to lower their prices due to increased veterinary competition in their area. Several pet owners look for the cheapest services available as every third reason of changing a practice is the price of services. Contradictorily, pet owners place service prices on the ninth rank when asked for the 12 most important factors for their veterinary practice choice. Price hikes of more than 20% will lead to a loss of more than 40% of clients whereby especially the lower-income groups of clients will react negatively to a greater extent [2].

The pricing structure for services is not as easy as for products as e.g. prescriptions only medicines can be priced with a mark-up of 50-100% whereas the mark-up ranges of pharmacy and merchant items should be lower [11]. Services can only be defined as an average as there are massive time variations depending on the case or the consulting veterinarian. In any case, the budget needs to be covered by the service fees. Different strategies can be used for pricing including the addition of X% to the last year's fees, cost plus X% and cost centre analysis [11]. Another approach is the market-driven approach for pricing [11].

This fee calculation can be translated in three different ways of service fee pricing being the fixed-price, time-based or menu price system. In many practices, the service fees are fixed as a basic fee and can be adjusted depending on the actual time spent for the procedure. Moreover, the number of animals can be also taken into consideration with fees going down with increasing patients' number of the same owner. In many practices, a variation of both choices is usually applied [11].

In some countries like Germany, fixed prices for veterinary services have been set up in a special veterinary fee structure which is mandatory for veterinarians. The fees can be raised up to the maximum three times depending on the location, purchase power of clients and difficulty of treatment. However, it is forbidden by law to raise prices above this fee structure or to price individually [9].

Due to the intensive competition of online veterinary shops, pricing of diet food, pet foods and prescription food is much more difficult to price as the mark-up ranges of internet suppliers are usually lower than in veterinary practices. It can help to follow the manufacturers' recommendation and to closely follow up price developments on the online shops.

Despite love to animals, a veterinarian and a veterinary practice has to survive as well. A good way is to find other alternatives, which might help in boosting the profit like new services or entirely different sources of income [6] like e.g. nutrition consultation. The newly introduced services like nutrition consultation in the veterinary practice might be causing low expenses but generate a high service volume. The high new service volume might translate into a good profit for the veterinary practice. Then the veterinary surgeon can evaluate if the newly introduced service of e.g. nutrition consultation is a valuable asset for the practice.

9.7. DECISION MAKING FOR CAPITAL INVESTMENTS

Capital investments, e.g. equipments, vehicles, computer hardware and software have to be well-thought before being purchased. The critical factor for the purchase decision is time as a considerable amount of cash money will be spent on the capital investment. Before buying capital items, it is advisable to evaluate the investment in terms of return on investment. Several evaluation methods exist for this purpose. In this chapter, we will focus on the most useful and practically used ones, the Net Present Value (NPV) and payback period (PP). When making new capital investment decisions, the practice owner or manager has to be aware of hidden costs of capital items. This means that the additional costs like fixed costs to operate the machine, salary of the person who operates it, insurance, and so on. On the other hand, the NPV shows benefits of the new investment like number of sales, money saved by using the new equipment and income through sales of the equipments in a few years [1].

Net Present Value

The Net Present Value calculation considers all costs for the capital investment as well as the time frame for costs and benefits. It is a very well leveraged method that poses most advantages for correct capital investment decision making [1].

Payback Period (PP)

The payback period is defined as "the length of time it takes for an initial investment to be repaid out of the cash inflows." [1, p.336]. The payback period has a maximum period in which the investment has to be paid back. Its duration makes the capital investment acceptable or not.

9.8. CONCLUSION

Financial management of the veterinary practice is very important as it helps to oversee and judge the financial performance of the business. Profit planning is one of the fields that require attention. For setting up a business plan, the break-even analysis is crucial and has to be studied very well in order to establish a successful and profitable business. Although this is often difficult for veterinarians in the beginning, the ratios can be broken down in profitability, efficiency and liquidity ratios. This helps to determine the status of the individual business areas. Pricing is another area that requires care and caution. If the prices at opening of a new veterinary practice were set up too low, it is very difficult to rise afterwards and will lead to massively reduced profitability or even loss. Capital investment has to be regarded as a high financial burden and needs to pay back in the fastest time possible.

REFERENCES

[1]   Atrill, P. and McLaney, E. (2006). Accounting and finance for non-specialists. 5th ed. Pearson Education LTd. Harlow. England.

[2]   Brown, J.P. and Silverman, J.D. (1999). The current and future market for veterinarians and veterinary medical services in the United States. *JAVMA,* Vol. 215, No. 2, July 15. pp. 161-183.

[3]   Ciancanelli, P., Dunn, J., Koch, B. and Stewart, M. (2006). Financial and management accounting. 4th ed. Glasgow: *The Graduate School of Business University of Strathclyde.*

[4]   CompanyRef (2007). Return on capital employed (ROCE). http://companyrefs.com/ Guide/keyROCE.htm (Accessed on January 20th, 2007).

[5]   Gillespie, A. (1998). *Advanced Business Studies through diagrams.* Oxford University Press. UK.

[6]   Megginson, W.L., Byrd, M.J. and Megginson, L.C. (2000). Small business management: An entrepreneur's guidebook. 3rd ed. McGraw-Hill. Boston, Madrid, Toronto.

[7]   Muller, M.G. (2007). Accounting. MBA Assignment.University of Strathclyde. *Graduate School of Business.* Glasgow, UK.

[8]   Nobes, C. (1995). The economist books: Pocket accounting. Penguin Group. Hamondsworth, Middlesex, England.

[9]   Ouwerkerk, M. and Schlegel, H. (1997). Erfolgreich Praxisfuehrung fuer den Tierarzt: Praxismanagament/ Praxismarketing. Hannover. Schluetersche GmbH.

[10]   Rutherford, B.A. (2002). Design and implementation of return on capital employed performance indicators within a trading regime: the case of executive agencies. Financial Accountability & management. Vol. 18, No. 1, pp.73-101. http://www.blackwell-synergy.com/doi/abs/10.1111/1468-0408.00146 (Accessed on January 21st , 2007).

[11]   Shilcock, M. and Stutchfield, G.(2008). Veterinary practice management. A practical guide. 2nd ed. Saunders, Elsevier Ltd. Philadelphia.

[12]   The Entrepreneur Magazine (1999). Small business advisor. 2nd ed. John Entrepreneur Media Inc. Wiley&Sons. New York, Chichester, Weinheim, Brisbane, Singapore, Toronto.

[13]   Wikipedia (2007). Return on capital employed. http://en.wikipedia.org/wiki/ Return_on_capital_employed (Accessed on January 20th, 2007).

Chapter 10

ADMINISTRATIVE MANAGEMENT

ABSTRACT

The smooth and efficient administration of the veterinary practice is vital for its success. The receptionist serves as the face of the practice to clients and the outside world. Therefore, a highly professional but personal and individual attendance of each client is a must for every successful veterinary practice. Waiting time can be drastically reduced through a well implemented appointment booking system. Online appointment bookings can ease pressure on the reception staff and enhance flexibility among the clients. This implies not only excellent receptionist skills, but phone manners as well. A modern telecommunication system with voice over helps to direct client inquiries to the right staff member. Either small or large veterinary practices can benefit from the introduction of an Authorities Matrix which states clearly the distribution of authorities among individual senior staff members and creates a strong framework of clear cut responsibilities. In this chapter, a sample appointment schedule and sample Authorities Matrix for a small and larger veterinary practice help to visualize those important topics.

10.1. INTRODUCTION

The administrative management of veterinary practices has changed tremendously in the past years with the introduction of veterinary practice managers in larger practices or veterinary hospitals. It is definitely required for modern practice management to have a sound knowledge of administrative and financial management.

The administrative management of veterinary practices comprises various areas like reception and appointment bookings, phone manners, procedures and policies for work of veterinary staff, administrative staff and laboratory staff. It also includes filing and archiving, duty rota schedules and vacation planning.

10.2. RECEPTION

The objectives that are expected by the work of receptionists are:

- Providing a very high level of professional service to the patient owners
- Providing professional and polite communication with pet owners
- Providing flawless phone manners and appointment scheduling
- Co-operating with all staff without bias at all times
- Efficiently and diligently performing their duties
- Enhancing one's knowledge by obtaining training
- Working accurately in order to avoid mistakes that may harm the veterinary practice's reputation

The reception of the veterinary practice is the first area the patient's owner will make contact with. It creates a lasting impression in the clients' mind. Clients, especially first-time clients, judge the whole hospital through the face of the practice, the receptionist. He/she is personifying the veterinary practice and therefore, relays the picture of the practice to the outside world. Therefore, the receptionist's performance is highly crucial to show a positive image to its customers.

The receptionist creates the first impression of the hospital and the care to be expected for both the owner and its falcon. He/she will also create the last impression everyone takes home with him when he is leaving the veterinary practice – this means the receptionist will create a lasting impression.

How does the veterinary practice want to be seen? This needs to spell out, not simply in terms of good medicine, professional patient care, efficient and high-quality staff – but also in terms of empathy, feelings, values as well as hospitable and courteous treatment.

10.2.1. Client Reception

As the veterinary practice is providing not only excellent medical care but also represents a place where friendly atmosphere and hospitality matters, it is expected that the patient owners, their family members and any other visitor are received with the due

- respect
- politeness
- courtesy
- professionalism and
- hospitality

As soon as the visitor enters the waiting room and comes to the reception, he will be politely greeted by the receptionist. In order to provide a customer-friendly environment in veterinary practices, it might be helpful to offer water, tea or coffee.

After completing the admission procedure the pet owner will be offered a seat in the waiting room and re-assured that he will be attended to as soon as possible. In modern veterinary practices, the separation of the waiting area into a cat and dog waiting area has proven to be very helpful and reduces stress for the pets and their owners alike. In cases of very large or aggressive dogs, it is advisable to let them wait outside the practice and to call them in only in time of their appointment.

If it is clear that the pet's owner may have to wait for a longer time due to unexpected emergencies or an extremely heavy patient flow, it is the receptionist's duty to inform him/her politely about the situation to avoid upsetting the client.

10.2.2. Appointment Bookings

It is advisable to introduce an appointment booking system for veterinary practices. This will lead to reduced waiting time and better work distribution and workflow among the staff members. As modern veterinary practices are supposed to have a well working website, a section for appointment bookings can be set up for online bookings. This reduces lost time for phone calls by the receptionist and easier appointment scheduling by customers. Each veterinarian should have his own appointment schedule that should not interfere in surgery times.

Another advantage of appointment schedules is the fact that patient details can be gathered before the actual visit and thus the daily work program of the veterinarian can be easier determined.

Below is a sample appointment schedule for three veterinarians who are working in different shifts and are divided between consultations and surgery. The sample plan is following the 20-minute appointment time for clients. Another possibility is 15 or 30 minutes per client [1]. However, the 20-minute time frame is convenient for the client and veterinarian as it provides sufficient time for a proper in-depth consultation and enough talking time to the clients.

Walk-in clients are accepted in many veterinary practices. However, animal owners with previous bookings have to be given preference to start the consultation at their scheduled time. In case of many bookings, walk-in clients have then to wait until a free slot is available.

10.2.3. Admission

For first-time pet owners, full details including Name, complete address, email, mobile number, office contact number has to be recorded. A consent form is advisable in order to protect the veterinary practice from liabilities.

If this pet is first-time patient, the following data have to be recorded on the patient admission sheet:

- species
- breed
- gender
- color
- date of birth
- microchip number
- tattoo
- last vaccination date
- vaccination reminder preferred

- previous diseases
- medications
- neutered
- allergies if known

In case of an already implanted microchip, the chip should be read and then registered.

If the pet has already been treated in the veterinary practice before, its file has to be taken out of the filing cabinet and forwarded to the veterinary nurse taking the patient to the examination room. The same applies to computerized files of veterinary software systems. In those cases, the nurse can already open the patient's file in the computer before the clients enter the consultation room. This gives the veterinarian time to review the previous visit and patient's history, if required.

Table 10.1. Sample appointment schedule

Time	Veterinarian 1	Veterinarian 2	Veterinarian 3
AM	+Nurse 2	+Head nurse	+ Assistant nurse
8.00-8.20	Ms. Smith, 1 dog, vaccination	Mrs. Anders	Off duty
8.20-8.40	Mr. Simons, 1 cat, not eating well	1 dog tooth extraction + dental cleaning	Off duty
8.40-9.00	Mr. Hurt, 1 dog, limping right hind leg	Mrs. Smithson 1 dog	Off duty
9.00-9.20	Mrs. Smith, 2 cats, sneezing	cruciate ligament	Off duty
9.20-9.40	Mr. Bond, 3 dogs, vaccination	surgery	Off duty
9.40-10.00	Ms. Saunders, 1 cat, pregnancy test		Off duty
10.00-10.20	Ms. Meyer, 1 cockatoo, not eating		Mrs. Ashman, 2 African grey parrots, nail + feather clipping
10.20-10.40	Coffee break	Coffee break	Mr. Porter, 1 dog, vaccination
10.40-11.00	Ms. Young, 1 tortoise, problem with carapax	Mr. Carter, 1 cat ulna fracture right	Ms. Richmond, 1 dog + 1 cat vaccination
11.00-11.20	Mr. Jones, 1 snake, lethargy		Mrs. York, 2 cats eye problems
11.20-11.40	Mrs. Jennings, 2 cats, vaccination		Mrs. Winter, 4 puppies, vaccination
11.40-12.00	Mrs. Norman, 1 dog, diarrhea		Mrs. Jones, 2 rabbits, coughing
PM			
12.00-12.20	Mrs. Vine, 1 dog, recheck pregnancy		Mr. Adams, 1 guinea pig, diarrhea
12.20-12.40	Ms. Sue, 1 cat + 6 kitten, recheck	Mr. Muller 1 cat, spaying	Mrs. Batterfield, 3 turtles, not well
12.40-1.00	Mrs. Watson, 1 dog, last pregnancy check	Mrs. Blair 1 cat Spaying	Mr. Kindle, 1 dog, health certificate
1.00-1.20	Lunch break	Lunch break	Ms. Birbeck, 2 ferrets, skin problems
1.20-1.40			Ms. Lopez, 1 parrot, not singing anymore

Time	Veterinarian 1	Veterinarian 2	Veterinarian 3
AM	+Nurse 2	+Head nurse	+ Assistant nurse
1.40-2.00			Mrs. Adelaide, 1cat + 3 kitten, check up
2.00-2.20	Mrs. Cassins, 1 dog, recheck fracture	Mr. Sarandon, 1 cat bulbus extirpation	Lunch break
2.20-2.40	Mrs. Turner, 1 dog, not walking anymore		
2.40-3.00	Mrs. Redford, 1 chinchilla, hair problem		
3.00-3.20	Mrs. Hutchins, 1 rabbit, cutting teeth	Mr. Bradfield, 1 dog, spaying	Mr. Muller, 1 dog, hip problem
3.20-3.40	Mrs. Temple, 2 rabbits, ear mites		Mr. Meyers, 1 cat, vomiting
3.40-4.00	Mrs. Madson, 5 puppies, vaccination+ deworming		Mrs. Butler, 2 cats, sneezing + coughing
4.00-4.20	Mr. Tinsall, 1 dog, skin problem	Mr. Sasson, 1 dog Neutering	Mrs. Reid, 1dog, bad breath from mouth
4.20-4.40	Mr. Benning, 2 dogs, recheck castration		Mr. King, 3 canaries, not well
4.40-5.00	Mrs. Dennis, 2 hamsters, not well	Ms. Patterson, 1 cat, spaying	Coffee break
5.00-5.20	Off duty	Off duty	Not booked yet
5.20-5.40			Ms. Newman, 2 guinea pigs, not well
5.40-6.00			Mr. Wallis, 1 cat, swelling on leg
6.20-6.40			Mrs. Aniston, 1 dog, back problem
6.40-7.00			Not booked yet
7.00-7.20			Not booked yet
7.20-7.40			Mrs. Robinson, 1 dog, limping
7.40-8.00			Mr. Pierre, 1 cat, fallen from tree

10.2.4. Discharge

The receptionist responsible for discharging the patients has to check the computerized files or hard copy file for complete details of the visit and entered services. He will remind the client again of the medication plan. In case of a recheck appointment, he arranges the appointment with the client immediately.

After billing, the receptionist will give an invoice to the client and receipt after receiving the payment. One invoice and receipt copy will be retained in the patient's file. Before the owner leaves the receptionist checks the vaccination dates and asks the owner, whether he would like to be reminded when the next vaccination is due. He then enters the data in the vaccination database.

Pending cases, e.g. with pending laboratory results will be placed in the doctors' pending folder. Finished cases will be returned to the filing cabinet after all required copies have been taken out and distributed to the relevant department (administration, finance, etc.). In case of a fully computerized veterinary hospital management system, this will be updated automatically. In case of a separate check out billing counter, the invoicing procedure as part of the finance department and will be performed by the accountant responsible.

10.3. TELECOMMUNICATIONS

A very useful tool for efficient administrative management and client satisfaction is the Voice over IP (VOIP). It is a relatively new technology that works through phone calls via the internet [2]. All different types of communication like data, voice and multimedia can be put together in one single network. Despite initial higher investment costs, VOIP can save up to 50% costs compared to a separate voice and data system [2]. Other advantages include the so-called click-to-call. The caller can use the number from an onscreen directory or spoken after the first dial tone. It is very easy to forward calls to other people even in different locations [2]. These features greatly enhance client satisfaction and reduce the number of call at the reception. VOIP leads to unified messages as e-mails, voice mails and faxes are integrated in one single inbox [2]. Conference calls are possible as well as hot-desking which is the opportunity to access call by logged in staff, whether being on-site or off-site. With regard to costs, VOIP leads to greater transparency and cost control as all costs can be allocated and reviewed between the different business units [2].

Voice or IP can be implemented by using the existing telephone system and upgrading it to VOIP [2]. This is usually a very practical approach for already established veterinary practices.

Another possibility is to replace all telephone systems completely which can be costly and disruptive [2]. However, for new or relocating practices this can be a very cost-efficient solution. Hosted services through application providers are another choice to implement VOIP. Although cost-efficient, there might be a concern regarding the potential outsourcing of the entire phone directory to the provider [2].

Peer-to-peer solution can be used for introducing VOIP such as Skype, which has several options like Skype Voicemail, SkypeIn and SkypeOut. SkypeOut is very user-friendly for smaller businesses as it reduces the costs of 1 phone or mobile calls compared to traditional billing [2].

10.4. PHONE MANNERS

Successful telephone communication follows some basic rules. Whatever phone call any staff member makes or whatever phone call they receive, making this voice-only communication successful is dependent on the following four underlying factors:

- The basic rules of telephone communication
- How to use the voice
- The use of language
- Listening

10.4.1. Basic Rules of Telephone Communication

Some basic rules of telephone communication can make a major difference in client management and tremendously enhance client satisfaction. They make the difference between an average veterinary practice and an excellent veterinary practice.

Answer Promptly
A prompt answer is mandatory as anything else shows inefficiency. Four rings are universally recommended as the maximum time before picking up the telephone.

Identify Yourself
It is not sufficient to say a mere hallo. The receptionist identifies the organization and himself by answering the phone with the polite phrase: "Happy Veterinary Practice, ……… speaking, good morning" or in the afternoon: "Happy Veterinary practice, ……… speaking, good afternoon". The next phrase has to welcome the caller by asking "How may I help you?".

Hold the Phone Correctly
This seems to be an obvious rule but is often underestimated and neglected. However, it does affect hearing if the receiver is tucked under the chin or pushed aside as the staff on the phone may reach for something. Every staff member on the phone must be clearly audible.

Transfer Calls that Are Not Meant for the Reception
Calls from patient owners for the doctor conducting the treatment or any other staff member should be transferred in a friendly manner by telling the client: "I will transfer you to ……" or "May I transfer you to ……" in case the problem cannot be handled by the person answering the phone call.

Adopt an Appropriate Manner
This is not a question of insincerity or acting. However, good and attentive staff may want to emphasize certain traits more with some people that with others such as:

- an efficient-sounding yet friendly tone,
- a friendly, yet firm one with those causing trouble
- a compassionate tone with those whose favorite pet had to be put down or is critically ill.

Listen Carefully
The telephone is a voice-only medium, but it is also two-way. It is important not to do all the talking as this is the only way to extract information from the caller. Listen carefully to what the client wants and needs to know. Furthermore, it is wise to make accurate notes. A good gesture to make clear that somebody is listening can be repeating the most important points.

Be Polite

A L W A Y S (even if the client or whoever is on the other side of the line is rude) be polite! It is absolutely important to maintain reasonable courtesies, and with voice only, it can be easy to sound rude when you are trying to speed things up or the client is calling for the same issue a lot of times. If the caller is ill-mannered and impolite, it is still required to stay calm and polite but firm. Voice can display such emotions and therefore, helps to calm the caller down and put him in his place.

Have the Right Information to Hand

Many calls involve repetitive elements. The receptionist or any staff members will make calls and their life a lot easier when they are well-organized and have the information needed to hand.

Take Care with Names, Phone Numbers and Addresses

People are sensitive about their names. Get them right – do so early-on– ask for the spelling, if pronounced unclear. Always ask for the mobile phone contact number, as these numbers may change. Always ask for the complete address as the administration and the veterinary side will need this information. If the receptionist does not consider this as an important piece of information he will create a lot of unnecessary work for his colleagues and therefore take away their time from doing their job.

Take Care with the Microchip or Other Identification Number

As all patients are identified with a microchip number, tattoo or ring number, those have to be checked and verified. It is imperative to take great care when noting these numbers down as they determine which patient is inquired for. There is no greater embarrassment for all staff members when they have to talk about a patient health status to anyone but the owner by mistake.

10.4.2. Using Voice to Positive Effect

Few of the techniques referred to so far will work well without consideration of that most important element of the telephone manners: the voice.

Not only is the voice an important element, it has to act alone: by definition telephone communication is voiced- only. As with the basic rules, detail here matters. The following, in no particular order of priority are all important:

Speak at an Appropriate Pace

Speaking at an appropriate pace should not be overdone and to slow down to such an extent that the person on the phone appears to be half a-s-l-e-e-p. But pace is important. A considered pace is more likely to allow things to be made clear, and misunderstandings to be avoided. It allows the listener to keep up, particularly, for example, when clearly they may want to make a note: slow down especially for that.

Smile

Even though a smile cannot be seen, a pleasant smile produces a pleasant tone with the right sound. A warm tone of voice produces a feeling that the speaker is pleasant, efficient, helpful and, most importantly, interested in the person at the other end.

Ensure Clarity

It is not sounding pleasant if what the person on the phone says cannot be understood. Be clear; be particularly careful about names, numbers, diagnosis and dates.

Be Concise

Most people you will speak with expect and appreciate you respecting their time. This means your message should be concise and precise. "I think" or "I guess" should not be used at all. If you do not know the answer, then it is advisable to transfer politely the caller to the person in command.

10.4.3. Listening

Good communications demand excellent listening skills. This is especially important on the telephone when there are few other signs. Not only does it give you more information, other people feel well treated. However, the ability to listen properly does very rarely come by itself; it usually requires hard work to achieve it.

Want to Listen

This is easy once you understand how useful it is.

Sound Like a Good Listener

This comes through both the language when using phrases like "tell me about... (symptoms, time these symptoms occur, are other pets affected, does the cat/dog have other problems)" and tone.

React

Let the caller know you are listening by making small acknowledging comments – "right", "I understand", "we will try to help your pet".

Stop Talking

Remember, you cannot talk and listen at the same time, nor it is polite to try to do so. By stopping to talk, you give the caller the chance to express himself and explain issues more detailed.

Use Empathy

Put yourself in the caller's shoes and make you appreciate their worry, concern and point of view.

10.5. FILING

Filing as such is designed to store all information, to be accessed easily and provide a proper archive for the data processed. A comprehensive, efficient and simple filing system has to be established soonest to cater for the need of both the administrative and veterinary part of the practice.

Currently the receptionists have to ensure as their responsibility

- that files are stored properly in the filing cabinet,
- that files are found swiftly
- that the file content is complete.

It is unacceptable to

- search for one single file for hours,
- have pile of file in one corner somewhere in the administrative part of the practice
- to set up several files for the identical patient
- not being able to find the file needed at all.

Nowadays, more and more veterinary practices use computerized filing system and patient dossiers. Despite the advantage of having all information available in different work stations at the same time and the reduction of paper, a computer breakdown might lead to loss of data and delay to recover patient information. It is inevitable to have good back up taking of computerized files in place.

10.6. DELEGATION OF AUTHORITIES

The delegation of authorities through the Authorities Matrix establishes the basis of authorization and accountability for the veterinary practice management to commit resources or incur liabilities or obligations. This is especially helpful in larger practices or corporate veterinary practice groups. However, the delegation of authorities can be also used in smaller practices to clarify responsibilities of practice owner and staff.

10.6.1. General Information to Authorities' Matrix

An Authorities Matrix contains the delegation of authorities of critical business areas. It helps to support the well-defined decision-making process in a number of important business areas for the veterinary practice [3]. Therefore, the Authorities Matrix provides a clear-cut framework for all staff that enables them to act instantly in their delegated responsibilities or to address a person with higher authority. This helps to save time and enhances the self-confidence of staff as they know to whom to go with certain issues. Each Authorities Matrix has to be communicated to the staff to make them aware of it. It is good to integrate senior practice staff in establishing the matrix as this will foster their buy-in. Additionally, the

Authorities Matrix reflects the roles and responsibilities and reporting lines as per both the agreed corporate governance framework and organization structure for the veterinary practice. It should be viewed as a tool that supports the implementation of good corporate governance practices [3]. The Authorities Matrix is intended to supplement existing operating policies. Although it might look a bit complicate in the beginning, the Authorities Matrix will be set up only once and then just reviewed annually or as and when needed. Compliance with the authority levels set forth in the delegation of Authorities Matrix should be reviewed regularly (at least annually) as part of the internal audit activities [3].

There are three different types of authorities depicted in the Authorities Matrix:

- *First stage*: Recommend (RC): The authority to initiate or propose an action, task, idea or plan and recommend the outcome for approval. The next stage in the decision making process is the review stage [3].
- *Second stage*: Review (RV): The authority to consider and assess a presented recommendation and any related information pertaining to a certain decision, and put forward views and position to the decision making authority. The review is normally performed against the veterinary practice's strategy, plans, and objectives, set policies and procedures, risks and envisioned benefits as applicable. The next and final stage in the decision making process is the approval stage [3].
- *Third stage*: Approve (AP): The authority to sanction a decision for implementation or adoption [3].

10.6.2. Authorities Matrix for a Small Veterinary Practice

Small veterinary practices consist mainly of the veterinary practice owner who works as the head veterinarian, another veterinary surgeon or assistant veterinarian, nursing and reception staff. The main responsibilities lay on the practice owner with a delegation of some authorities to the next senior veterinarian and the head nurse. Often, an external Certified Public Accountant (CPA) is used to support the financial side of the veterinary practice. Although not being practice staff, the Certified Public Accountant has a function in the overall Authorities Matrix and should be included in its financial part. The samples table for small veterinary practices cannot consider each single detail, but is intended to give an overview of the different level of authorities. The final decision of authorities' levels solely depends on the practice owner who in the case of a small veterinary practice naturally holds most of the authorities.

Table 10.2. Sample Authorities Matrix for a small veterinary practice (PO=Practice owner, V=Veterinarian, HN=Head Nurse, CPA=Certified Public Accountant) [modified from 3 for veterinary practice]

Activity	PO	V	HN	Others
1. Strategy and business planning				
1.1 Vision, mission, values	AP/RV	RV		
1.2. Business strategy, 3 years business plan	AP/RV	RV		

Table 10.2. (Continued)

Activity	PO	V	HN	Others
1.3. Annual plan and budget	AP/RV	RV		RC (CPA)
1.4. Financial commitment of more than 100,000 US$	AP/RV			RC (CPA)
2. Governance				
2.1.Changes to corporate governance structure	AP	RC		
2.2. Changes in policies and procedures	AP	RC		
2.3. Appointment of external auditors	AP			RV (CPA)
2.4.Approval of audited financial statements	AP/RV			RV (CPA)
3. Operation				
3.1. Submission, review and approval of Standard Operating Procedures (SOPs)	AP/RV	AP/RV	RC	
3.2. Interaction with press, media, radio	AP	AP/RV	RC	
3.3. Submission, review and approval of public lectures	AP	AP/RV	RV/RC	
3.4. Selection of IT system	AP	RV/RC	RC	
3.5.IT policies and procedures	AP	RV/RC	RC	
4. Procurement				
4.1. Approval purchase order within budget				
Capex/Opex				
Up to 10,000 US$	AP	AP	RV	
Above 10,000 and up to 100,000 US$	AP	RV		
Above 100,000 US$	AP/RV	RC		
4.2. Procurement policies and procedures				
5. Finance				
5.1. Non budgeted items				
Capex/Opex				
Up to 10,000 US$	AP	RC		RV (CPA)
Above 10,000 and up to 100,000 US$	AP	RC		RV (CPA)
Above 100,000 US$	AP/RV	RC		RV (CPA)
5.2. Disposal of capital assets				
Up to 10,000 US$	AP	RC		RV (CPA)
Above 10,000 and up to 100,000 US$	AP	RC		RV (CPA)
Above 100,000 US$	AP	RC		RV (CPA)
6. Accounts / banks				
6.1. Approval of quarterly accounts reports	AP			RC (CPA)
6.2. Approval of year end extraordinary adjustments	AP			RV (CPA)
6.3. Opening of bank account	AP			
7. Authorized signatures	AP			
7.1. Cheque signing	AP			

Activity	PO	V	HN	Others
8. Marketing				
8.1. Marketing and branding strategy	AP	RV/RC	RC	
8.2. Initiatives, campaigns, advertisement, etc.	AP	AP/RV	RV/RC	
9. Manpower planning				
9.1. Manpower planning	AP	RV/RC	RC	
9.2. Organization structure and chart	AP	RV/RC	RC	
9.3. Establish job descriptions and evaluations	AP	RV/RC	RC	
9.4. Approval of employment offers and contracts	AP			
9.5. Confirmation of satisfactory completion of probationary period	AP	RV/RC		
9.6. Change of employee status	AP	RV/RC		
9.7. Amendments of employee contracts	AP	RV/RC		
9.8. Overtime	AP	RV/RC		
9.9. Leave (annual, sick, maternity, exam, etc.)	AP	RV/RC		
9.10. Salary structure	AP	RC		
9.11. Bonus payment	AP	RC		
9.12. Promotion	AP	RC		
9.13. Disciplinary measures	AP			
9.14. Termination/approval of resignation	AP			
10. Others				
10.1. Inventory write off	AP	RV		RV (CPA)

Table 10.3. Sample Authorities Matrix for a large veterinary practice with practice manager (PO=Practice owner, PM=Practice Manager, HV=Head Veterinarian, HN=Head Nurse, FM= Finance Manager, HRM=Human Resources Manager) [modified from 3 for veterinary practice]

Activity	PO	PM	HV	HN	FM/HRM
1. Strategy and business planning					
1.1 Vision, mission, values	AP	RV	RC		
1.2. Business strategy, 3 years business plan	AP	RV	RV		
1.3. Annual plan and budget	AP	RV	RC		RC (FM)
1.4. Financial commitment of more than 100,000 US$	AP	RV			RC (FM)
2. Governance					
2.1.Changes to corporate governance structure	AP	RV/RC	RC		
2.2. Changes in policies and procedures	AP	RV/RC	RV/RC	RC	
2.3. Appointment of external auditors	AP	RC			RV (FM)
2.4.Approval of audited financial statements	AP	RV			RV (FM)
3. Operation					
3.1. Submission, review and approval of Standard Operating Procedures (SOPs)		AP/RV	AP/RV	RC	
3.2. Interaction with press, media, radio		AP	AP/RV	RC	

Table 10.3. (Continued)

Activity	PO	PM	HV	HN	FM/HRM
3.3. Submission, review and approval of public lectures		AP	AP/RV	RV/RC	
3.4. Selection of IT system		AP	RV/RC	RC	
3.5.IT policies and procedures		AP	RV/RC	RC	
4. Procurement					
4.1. Approval purchase order within budget Capex/Opex					
Up to 10,000 US$		AP	AP	RV	
Above 10,000 and up to 100,000 US$		AP	RV		
Above 100,000 US$	AP	RV	RC		
4.2. Procurement policies and procedures					
5. Finance					
5.1. Non budgeted items Capex/Opex					
Up to 10,000 US$		AP	RC		AP (FM)
Above 10,000 and up to 100,000 US$	AP	RV	RC		RV (FM)
Above 100,000 US$	AP	RV	RC		RV (FM)
5.2. Disposal of capital assets					
Up to 10,000 US$		AP	RC		AP (FM)
Above 10,000 and up to 100,000 US$	AP	RV	RC		RV (FM)
Above 100,000 US$	AP	RV	RC		RV (FM)
Activity	PO	PM	HV	HN	FM/HRM
6. Accounts / banks					
6.1. Approval of quarterly accounts reports		AP			AP (FM)
6.2. Approval of year end extraordinary adjustments		AP			AP (FM)
6.3. Opening of bank account		AP			AP (FM)
7. Authorized signatures	AP	AP			AP (FM, HRM)
7.1. Cheque signing (depending on amount)	AP	AP			AP (FM)
8. Marketing					
8.1. Marketing and branding strategy		AP	RV/RC	RC	
8.2. Initiatives, campaigns, advertisement, etc.		AP	AP/RV	RC	
9. Manpower planning					
9.1. Manpower planning		AP	RC	RC	RV/RC (HRM)
9.2. Organization structure and chart	AP	RV	RC	RC	RV/RC (HRM)
9.3. Establish job descriptions and evaluations			RV?RC	RC	AP (HRM)
9.4. Approval of employment offers and contracts		AP			RV/RC (HRM)
9.5. Confirmation of satisfactory completion of probationary period			RV/RC	RC	AP (HRM)
9.6. Change of employee status		AP	RC		AP/RV (HRM)
9.7. Amendments of employee contracts		AP	RV/RC		AP/RV (HRM)

Activity	PO	PM	HV	HN	FM/HRM
9.8. Overtime			RV/RC	RC	AP (HRM)
9.9. Leave (annual, sick, maternity, exam, etc.)			RV/RC		AP (HRM)
9.10. Salary structure	AP	RV	RC		RV/RC (HRM)
9.11. Bonus payment	AP	RV	RC		RV/RC (HRM)
9.12. Promotion		AP	RC		RV/RC (HRM)
9.13. Disciplinary measures			RV/RC	RC	AP/RV (HRM)
9.14. Termination/approval of resignation		AP			RV/RC (HRM)
10. Others					
10.1. Inventory write off		AP	RC		AP/RV (FM)

10.6.3. Authorities Matrix for a Larger or Group Veterinary Practice

With the introduction of the new job practice manager, the roles and responsibilities change in the veterinary practice. The responsibilities are now shared between the practice owner for more strategic and overall decisions and the practice manager for day to day work.

The same applies also to larger corporate group practices with dedicated finance and administration departments and their respective managers.

Such practices can contain special human resources managers who hold the responsibility for all staff related issues. The level of authorities often depends on financial amounts as well as staff positions and grades. The samples table for larger veterinary practices cannot take into consideration each single detail, but provides an overview of the level of authorities. The final decision of authorities' levels solely depends on the practice owners or the corporate group owners.

10.7. CONCLUSION

Due to structural changes in veterinary practices, the administration has to be adjusted to the new modern practice management. However, no matter what changes do arise, the reception is still the face to the client and gives the first positive or negative impression of the veterinary practice. Therefore, reception staff has to be trained especially well as mistakes can be fatal and lead to the loss of clients and thus income and profit. Both, client reception and appointment bookings can be critical to the veterinary practice's success. Personal and individual attention of the client by receptionist, nurse and veterinary surgeon alike hold the key to a good impression of the veterinary practice. This includes not only fast and efficient admission and discharges but also phone manners. Being often underestimated and neglected, phone manners can even influence the decision of a client to visit a veterinary practice or to choose another one. Modern telecommunication tools can help to support clients' expectations of picking up each single phone call immediately and to redirect them to the concerned practice staff member. Correct and immediate filing or entering in the veterinary practice software enables a smooth and faultless dealing with clients.

Although the idea of establishing an Authorities Matrix is a new feature in the veterinary practice administration, it is a highly useful tool of distributing responsibilities and delegating them to different levels. However, the delegation of authorities depends strongly on the size and structure of the veterinary practice or hospital as well as the number of senior administrative and finance staff members.

The final levels of authorities' delegations depend on the practice owners' idea of how to run the practice. Whereas often in small veterinary practices the owner is involved in each or almost each single decision-making process, this concept is not viable anymore in larger practices with several branches or corporate group practice. They function much more as business entities with different sub business units respectively branches. Consequently, this development has a major impact on the Authorities Matrix through stronger delegation of authorities.

REFERENCES

[1] Ackermann, Lowell (2007). Blackwell's five-minute veterinary practice management consult. *Blackwell Publishing.* Iowa. USA.

[2] Bocij, P., Chaffey, D., Greasley, A. and Hickie, S. (2006). Business information systems. Technology, development & management for the e-business. 3rd. ed. Prentice Hall. Financial Times.

[3] EAD (2010). Delegation of Authorities. *Environment Agency Abu Dhabi.* Abu Dhabi, UAE.

Chapter 11

CLIENT MANAGEMENT

ABSTRACT

Client management is one of the main pillars for successful veterinary practices. A good client management can contribute to the rapid growth of the practice and thus its profitability. Several problems can arise in the relationship between the client and veterinary practice employees which are highlighted in this chapter. New threats to client management have emerged lately with the wider distribution of competitive veterinary online pharmacies and veterinarians. This has led to a reduction of the practices' income and increased difficulties with the clients. Moreover, lack of compliance hampers proper patient care. Complaints are a usual feature in any veterinary practice and hospital. However, they need to be dealt with in an appropriate and professional way. Difficult clients are another problem that every veterinary practice has to face. This chapter details several kinds of different clients and offer solution to deal with them in the best way. A very good review of client satisfaction or dissatisfaction is the client satisfaction survey which is explained in detail in this chapter. If conducted on an annual basis, a large amount of information about the level of client satisfaction in various practice areas can be gathered and compared. Those trends lead to action plans with the aim to improve areas of greater dissatisfaction and to enhance excellence in the veterinary practice. All these tools lead to greater retention and satisfaction of clients and subsequently to increased income and profitability.

11.1. INTRODUCTION

Excellent client management is the most important success factor for the veterinary practice. It does not help if the professional work of the veterinary staff is outstanding but the profit and customer loyalty declines due to miserable and careless client care. Veterinary personnel have to be trained in the best way possible to serve their clients. Clients who do not feel well-received and well-treated might not only complain but also leave the practice and make poor propaganda about it. Complaints will always arise but have to be dealt with in a fast and efficient way. Not all complaints are justified and can be solved, but it is essential to let the complaining client understand that his concerns are taken care of. Another important issue in client management is the management of difficult clients, which exist in every veterinary practice. A helpful tool in understanding clients' opinions and conceptions about the veterinary practice are customer surveys. They aim at providing information and data about the clients as well as their view of the veterinary practice work. Client Satisfaction Surveys that are conducted over the period of several years will provide valuable information about trends that can positively or negatively affect the veterinary practice or hospital. The use of the terms "customer" has person buying products and "client" purchasing services is not so strict anymore and can be interchanged.

11.2. EXPECTATION OF CLIENTS

Veterinary practices need to understand the expectations of its clients in order to serve them in the best way possible. Nowadays, client expectations are ever increasing [5]. Veterinary practices and hospitals have to put much more efforts to meet and exceed the clients' expectation [5]. But what do clients expect?

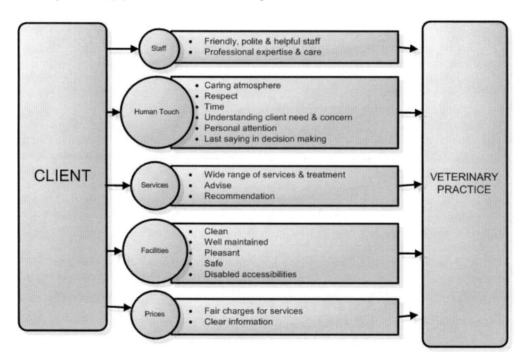

Figure 11.1. Client expectations.

Clients have an expectation in different areas among them the expectation of staff, human touch, services, facilities and pricing. Staff is expected to be welcoming, polite, helpful and courteous at all times. They should have the professional expertise and care to perform the best services and treatments for the animal. This is called "compliance" which is discussed later in this chapter in detail.

The human touch of the veterinary practice is one of the main areas that makes the difference between a good and poor veterinary practice. It reflects tremendously on the client and for this reason the clients' expectations are very high. Animal owners do not just only want a caring and welcoming practice atmosphere but also expect to be treated with respect.

They regard time for their and their pet's need as utmost important and do not appreciate long waiting times. Understanding the clients' needs, requirements and concerns are crucial to fulfill their expectation. Personal attention is highly critical to clients because this factor shows them that they are valued clients. Moreover, animal owners expect to have the last saying in the decision-making for their animals. They own the animal and will act on its behalf. Although veterinarians might not always agree with their decision, clients are right to expect that they have the ultimate right to decide.

Clients expect a wide range of services and treatments to get the best for their animal. They are also looking for advice and competent guidance by the practice team. Animal owners have an expectation with regard to facilities, too. This includes that facilities should be always clean and well-maintained. Pricing is another field where clients hold expectations. They wish for a fair charge of services rendered by the veterinary practice or hospital. Moreover, they prefer to get clear pricing information before services are undertaken and at least estimates for larger and costlier surgical interventions.

11.3. RELATIONSHIP CLIENTS – VETERINARY STAFF

The relationship between the veterinary practice and its personnel and the client starts already before the client enters the practice building physically. It begins with the first telephone call of the client to make an inquiry or appointment booking. If the client does not get his phone call answered he will get a negative impression about the veterinary practice right from the start. The first physical contact being the first visit of the veterinary practice determines the client – veterinary staff relationship to a great deal. Apart from the fact that the receptionist has to be friendly, courteous and polite to every client, there is still the element of sympathy and antipathy between people when they first meet. This applies also to the receptionist when seeing the client. A professional receptionist will be able to handle the encounter with the new client in a perfect way. However, a not fully trained receptionist might be a bit tougher with the client if he dislikes him. As clients are sometimes very sensitive and stressed out when they enter the veterinary practice due to their sick animal, they can feel invisible vibrations stronger as this would normally be the case. Professional behavior of receptionists has been described in detail in the chapter 10 "Administrative Management" in this book.

The relationship between the veterinary nursing staff is often the next step in the pyramid of clients and practice personnel. Veterinary nurses have to be very dedicated and compassionate when dealing with pet owners. The way how they deal with the animal is critical to the owner's eye. Veterinary nurses have to be friendly to the client but must show their caring abilities to the animal in order to convince the client. In cases of already known patients, this can be achieved by a caring "how is Snoopy doing today?" instead of a rude "how is your dog today?". Animal owners are very sensitive about the way how their animal is dealt with.

For veterinary surgeons, it is highly critical to build a long-lasting relationship to the pet owners and to earn their trust. This cannot be done alone through professional expertise but through the right way of talking to clients and establishing a strong confidence in his work. This will inevitably lead to a loyal clientele. It should be kept in mind that it is the way how things are said and not always the content of what is said that makes the big difference in relations. Apart from professional expertise and work performance, honesty and integrity are important pillars to gain and keep the faith of pet owners. In almost every client and veterinary surgeon relation, the day will come when difficult decisions have to be taken, may it be a major surgical intervention or euthanasia of the pet. This is the time when this relationship will be tested. Only when the client trusts the veterinary practitioner to a hundred percent, this decision will be taken in the interest of all in a timely manner.

The veterinary practice owners or managers might have a slightly different relationship with pet owners. They often have to enforce existing rules, regulation and internal policies, especially when it comes to complaining clients and clients who would like to bypass the rules. In those cases, it is best to be firm but polite and to stick to the rules. There are clients who are trying to create extra rules and regulations. If successful, they will try to do it again and jump over the rules. Besides they will communicate their success to other clients who then will try to follow this example. Therefore, it is advisable to have the same rules for all in order to prevent such negative impact on the veterinary practice. If an exception from rules is made, a valid reason should exist. Furthermore, those exemption should be made by the responsible person who has to be the veterinary practice owners, practice managers or authorized veterinary surgeon as they are ultimately responsible for it.

11.4. Threats to the Client – Veterinary Practice Relationship

When looking at the return rate of clients in veterinary practices, alarming results can be found. A staggering 38% of clients do not return to the veterinary practice after their first visit [3]. In addition, 68% of clients leave the practice because they feel they are not cared for enough and feel a lack of attention [3].

This relates again to problems with veterinary staff as well as uneducated team members. Moreover, other contributing factors are long waiting times, being rushed too much and pressured to buy items that the clients do not want. Another issue for leaving a veterinary practice is the inability of veterinary personnel to explain facts in a not understandable way [3]. A further 14% customers change to another practice due to an experience that was not satisfying [3].

Recently, the relationship between clients and veterinary practices started to change. This is mainly happening due to external competition of outside sources threatening the practice's income through loss of veterinary services or annual vaccination [3]. It is therefore very critical for the veterinary practice to determine the source of those losses [3] and to find counter strategies to preserve the practice's income.

Income and profit losses can be caused by external shops or the internet selling veterinary items and even veterinary medicines. Online veterinary pharmacies have become a major threat to traditional veterinary practices. People all over the world tend to get to the internet first to search information on any issue they are interested in. Nowadays, several online veterinary pharmacies in the United States, Canada and Europe offer identical products that the pet owners traditionally get from their veterinarians. They advertise those products to be sold at consistently low prices. This includes even prescription's products like anti-inflammatory medicines as well as vaccines. With regard to vaccines, an online veterinary pharmacy in the United States even actively supports to vaccine pets at home. It recommends vaccinating the pet at home because it is easier, saves time and is less expensive than taking it to the veterinarian.

In order to advise the online customers, they provide a video that shows how to give the vaccine injections. Apart from the fact that they undermine the use of the annual veterinary visit of not only administering the vaccine but also to conduct a yearly health check up of the animal, they remove regular income from the veterinary practice. If this example takes off in popularity, veterinary practices will face stiff competition, especially in economic difficult times and recession as well as among low income clients. With strong growth of online sales in all different fields and wider accessibility and use of the internet, it can be expected that online veterinary pharmacies will get a much higher market share soon.

Moreover, online veterinary shops and pharmacies offer a wide range of pet accessories like collar, leashes and dog food. These are all parts of additional income for the traditional veterinary practice and can sensitively affect the income and profit structure of the practice.

Another threat to the traditional veterinary practice is the online veterinarian consultation. With the internet usage, online veterinary consultations are on the rise. Well designed websites offer to answer pet owner questions within minutes. The payment fee is low and according to the advertisement only applicable in cases of answers that are satisfying to the customer.

One of those websites invites pet owners to join more than one million satisfied customers. Their veterinary experts have all more than 8-10 years professional experiences in various fields of small animal medicine. The positive customers' feedback for those experts exceeds 99% for each one of them. Although it cannot be verified if those numbers and information are really true, such websites can be definitely regarded as newly emerging competition for veterinary practices. And which veterinarian has not yet faced the comment of a client who said "but I have read in the internet that….".

Other new issues in the relationships between clients and the veterinary practice that arise with the wider distribution of the internet are blogs and internet discussion forums. Pet owners might have their own blogs nowadays where they comment on veterinary treatment and might comment about the veterinary practices and their services. If the comments are pleasant, it will be good for the veterinary practice. However, if the comments are negative and usually the tendency is that more unsatisfied clients will put their comments, it can have a massively negative impact on the reputation of the veterinary practice.

As the internet does still lack a legal framework, the veterinary practice can do little to rectify such comments. One way of counteracting is the use of a special veterinary practice blog with positive comments of clients on the practice website. Although veterinarian and their team are busily working, it might be worth checking the internet from time to time to detect such client blogs.

In future, such blogs and internet discussion forum will certainly increase and should be watched. The same applies to social media like Facebook, twitter and LinkedIn as especially younger people use those platforms frequently and even sometimes on a daily basis. Therefore, it can happen that pet owners post comments after the visit of their pet to the veterinary practice.

11.5. COMPLIANCE

Compliance is defined as "the extent to which pets receive a treatment, screening or procedure in accordance with accepted veterinary health care practices. Compliance involves both veterinary staff performing and/or recommending treatments, screenings and procedures *and* pet owner follow through." [2, p.1]. In contrast, adherence is "The extent to which patients take medication prescribed, involving the pet owner in filling and refilling the prescription; administering the correct dose, timing and use; and completing the prescribed course. Adherence is a term applied specifically to medications; it does not refer, for example, to recommendation for wellness check, diagnostic screenings and so on." [2, p1].

A first survey on compliance among American pet owners was conducted by the American Animal Hospital Association AAHA in 2002 [1]. It revealed alarming results about the massive lack of compliance. Non-compliance rates reached 82% for feline therapeutic diets and 81% for canine therapeutic diets. This was followed by 68% non-compliance in canine senior screening. Feline senior screening and dental prophylaxis reached both 65% non-compliance rates among pet owners followed by 13% in core vaccines [4]. The main reason for non-compliance among pet owners was that they did not understand the importance of the veterinarian's recommendations as the veterinary practitioners and their health care team failed in making effective recommendations [4]. Moreover, pet owners did complain about lacking recommendation's follow up. Another reason was that recommendations were made without helping the client to implement them at home [4]. As clients did not refuse the recommendation for cost reasons, it became clear that the lack of understanding was the main problem leading to non-compliance [4]. The study also showed that by many veterinary practitioners, compliance was overestimated by at least 25% [3]. Furthermore, 60% of veterinary professionals believed that compliance falls in the client's responsibility [2]. This massive lack of compliance does not only lead to reduced therapeutic care for pets and frustrated veterinary team members but results also in considerable loss of income for veterinary practices [4].

The comparative study by AAHA six years later showed major positive changes in perceptions and compliance rates. In the 2008 study, 60% of veterinary staff regarded compliance as the responsibility of the veterinary team and not the pet owner [2]. Moreover, the overall compliance rates improved from 64% to 73% with increases in all parameters except vaccines [2].

AAHA developed the "CRAFT" formula which can be summarized as follows:

Table 11.1. "CRAFT" formula [4, p.207]

C = R x A x F x T
C = Compliance
R = Recommendation by veterinarian and reinforced by healthcare team
A = Acceptance by client
FT = Follow through by veterinary healthcare team

This formula clearly shows that the major part of compliance lies in the hands of the veterinary team and not in the hands of the client.

The veterinary team [3]:

- Sets the compliance standards of care
- Makes the recommendation
- And provides the follow through by rechecks and revisits

The client is responsible for [3]:

- Accepting the recommendations

The veterinary team responsibilities are twofold. Firstly, the veterinary practitioner gives the clients the specific recommendation and treatment protocol. Secondly, the veterinary nurses and other team members have to reinforce actively this recommendation, e.g. by talking to the client about the given recommendation and explaining its importance. It is their job to help the clients to follow through the recommendation [4] and to follow up with them later by scheduling recheck appointments. The AAHA study stated a demand by 80% of pet owners to talk in-depth about their pet's care with veterinary team members like nurses and not only veterinary practitioners [4]. This shows the tremendous importance of well trained veterinary nursing staff in increasing pet owners' compliance with the veterinary recommendations.

Compliance levels can be actively raised by providing training to the veterinary staff members to enhance their effective communication skills. Such effective communication skills are manifold and include listening skills and improved empathy skills [4]. Communication is improved by better knowledge about services and products as well as using product samples, especially for prescription diets [4] and dental products. Veterinary personnel need to know how to clarify and support the veterinarian's recommendation. Furthermore, selling skills as well as improved merchandising skills and product display is another training area for veterinary health care staff [4].

However, not just compliance, but adherence to medication need to be increased. Adherence levels for improved use of prescribed medicine protocols can be raised by six important communication practices demonstration, length of appointments, written information, follow-up calls, chronic medication reminders and continuity with the veterinary practitioner [2]. These communication practices can be divided among team members as follows:

- Clear demonstration (firstly by the veterinarian and then reinforced by the veterinary nurses)
- Increased length of appointment (to be scheduled by the receptionist and to block veterinarian's time)
- Full detailed written information (either by special product information, leaflets produced internally in the practice for client use and or written by the veterinary nurse)
- Clearly scheduled follow-up calls (by the receptionist and veterinary nurse)
- Routine chronic medication reminders (by the receptionist upon information of the veterinarian)

- Continuity with the veterinarian (receptionist has to schedule appointments with the same veterinary practitioner)

Adherence level to prescribed medication can be further raised through medicines that are easy to administer. Pet owners are very much willing to pay even a higher price for medicines if they can give them to their pet in an easier way [2].

With increased levels of compliance, adherence as well as excellent veterinary teamwork and communication, a major improvement in patients' care can be achieved. This should be regarded as the ultimate aim of all compliance efforts.

11.6. COMPLAINT MANAGEMENT

Every veterinary practice will hear complaints even if it is the perfect practice. However, this does not say anything about the justification of the complaint. Complaints may be valid but can be also unjustified. The best way to find out about the reason and justification of the complaint is to listen to the person who complains. It is highly important to take each person who complains seriously as they will feel this and this will help to cool them down. Complaints can lead to detect problems in the veterinary services or staff and can provide a great opportunity to improve the veterinary practice. Although the saying "the customer is king" exists, it does not mean that the client is always right!

Every veterinary practice needs to have a proper complaint procedure in place [5]. The complaint procedure should have several levels of responsibilities in dealing with complaints. A small issue can be dealt with by the receptionist or the veterinary nurse. However, larger medical issues have to go back to the veterinary practitioner. Practice owners or practice managers are in command to handle very complex complaint or complaints of non veterinary nature [5] like administrative or invoicing complaints. A practice complaint procedure provides support and confidence to the veterinary team members as they understand their role and responsibility in complaint cases much clearer than without procedures. It gives the framework to pass the complaint to other responsible persons who might be equipped with more authority [5].

The best way of dealing with complaints is in a separate room as not all other clients need to hear about potential real or unreal problems in the veterinary practice. Then the client should be asked what he wants to complain about to get a full picture of the complaint issue. After he finishes, it is better to wait a few seconds before answering. The first best answer is to agree that the client is upset [3] which does not mean to agree to their complaint or to give in to it. This usually appeases the client at least to a certain extent. It now depends on the fact if the complaint is justified because the veterinary practice has made a mistake or something went wrong, or if it is unjustified and just a distorted perception of the client. In case of a justified complain or a mistake of the veterinary practice, the veterinary practitioner or responsible person has to apologize immediately because the client will not accept anything less. It is best to handle substantiated complaints in a quick and efficient way [5]. In contrast, an apology shows the client that the veterinary practice is able and serious about admit a mistake and is ready to rectify it. In such a case, a suitable compensation is required for example to give a free grooming for a wrong hair cut. Vouchers for discounted treatment or vaccination can help to compensate a complaining client [5]. However, in some cases the mistake cannot be reversed, and the responsible person has to find a way to compensate the pet owner.

The good news is that 95% of pet owners with complaints will stay as a client in the veterinary practice if their complaint is rectified immediately. Another 70% will remain at the veterinary practice if they realize that all efforts are undertaken to clear the complaint [5]. Therefore, fast and efficient complaint management is the key in the retention of complaining pet owners and turning them into happy clients.

11.7. DIFFICULT CLIENT MANAGEMENT

There is not one veterinary practice without difficult clients. Difficult clients might not be always a negative term, it can include a positive side, too. Most of the difficult clients may be nerve-racking clients but there are also very nice and sweet people. There exist several types of difficult clients.

The first category of difficult clients are sometimes clients who are just under personal stress or have stress in their jobs, which leads to mood swings. This so-called hidden agenda [5] can include worries about sick family members, problems to pay the house's mortgage, threatening unemployment or a bereavement. It is therefore essential for the receptionist and other practice team members to understand that a difficult client might be in an extraordinary personal situation that has nothing to do with the client's view of the practice staff.

The second group of difficult clients is the ones who are angry, never satisfied, rude and impolite to the practice staff and complaining about each and everything at every visit. Those clients can be really difficult to handle and pose a considerable challenge to the receptionist and veterinary team. They should be handled by more experienced staff with higher authority like the veterinarian or practice manager. In some cases, the veterinary practice will be left with only the choice to refuse to keep them as clients.

The third category of difficult clients is lonely or elderly people. These are mainly older ladies who live alone or a widowed and have nobody else than their beloved pet. They visit the veterinary practice frequently to come on people or call frequently for at least half an hour just for the sake of talking. These pet owners have often very nice and loving characters who will usually tell the story of their pet repeatedly. The main problem of those clients is mainly the time they consume. This can be helped by providing understanding for them and to integrate them in the practice workflow. As they often have a lot of time, they can wait in cases of unscheduled visits and talk with the other pet owners in the waiting room. This will give them the opportunity to highlight their beloved pet to other people and will make them tremendously proud of it. Another possibility of dealing with them is to return their call at a time when the practice is not too much frequented and the receptionist or nurse has more time. Such clients are good to keep as they can make a lot of positive mouth-to-mouth propaganda about the veterinary practice even in the waiting room.

Apart from really difficult clients, personal perceptions, especially by reception and nursing staff might lead to the creation of a demanding pet owner because they may not be able to cope with their character or way of talking. Sometimes even the external appearance leads to misperceptions among the receptionist and other veterinary team members. In such cases, only excellent staff training will help to avoid misperceptions. All practice staff have to be trained to be always polite, friendly, open and with positive attitude. If the receptionist is in a bad mood, how can we expect the client to be in a better mood? Therefore, veterinary practice staff has to be always attentive, controlling their mood and emotions and not fighting with clients. A nice smile helps often very much to appease difficult pet owners.

However, if nothing helps with the difficult clients, the veterinarian or practice manager must step in with authority and courage to deal with them in an appropriate way. This does not mean to shout at them but to tell them in absolutely clear words, and with particularly firm attitude that this is the end of the discussion and if the client does not comply with the practice's rules and regulations, he will not be accepted anymore as client and has to leave the practice. In some cases, the pet owner will relent and understand that he cannot go further. Usually, those clients change from a difficult to a normal client. In other cases, the client will leave the veterinary practice which should not be regarded as a loss.

11.8. CLIENT SATISFACTION SURVEY

11.8.1. Survey Preparation and Content

A client satisfaction survey in the form of a questionnaire should be performed on an annual basis. Its aim is to get feedback from customers of the veterinary practice and to obtain their opinions, ideas and views on practice's practice's role and how it can be enhanced to suit their needs. The survey serves as measurement of the current clients' satisfaction with the procedures of the veterinary practice. If conducted annually, the client satisfaction survey can compare satisfaction over the years and highlight areas of increased or decreased clients' satisfaction. This can be a helpful outcome for the practice to review problem areas and to introduce improvement measures.

Before being administered, the survey has to be planned carefully. It has to be decided of the size of the clients to be sampled and the time when it will be conducted. Depending on the size of the veterinary practice or hospital, a size of around 100 clients will provide strong information.

The size of the survey should be kept in a suitable range of a maximum 5-10 minutes answering time. Otherwise it takes too long, and clients will refuse to fill in the survey questionnaire questions. The questionnaire must have short and clear questions. Moreover, it has mostly closed ended and rating questions but a couple of open-ended questions are also included to get the clients' ideas and suggestions.

Survey questionnaire can be conducted face to face, which is the easiest and most effective way of getting the questionnaire answered completely. One member of the staff can be used to explain the reason for the survey and assist in filling it in. This is definitely the most recommended form of survey administration as it leads to the best and fastest results. Another possibility is the telephone survey which might be too much intruding in the customers' private sphere [5]. Handout questionnaires are given to the client in the reception, and he is supposed to complete it and return it directly to the receptionist. However, some clients do not have enough time as they might be called in the treatment room [5], are reluctant to fill the questionnaire or do not understand the reason for the survey.

Table 11.2. Sample Client Satisfaction Survey questionnaire

Happy Veterinary Practice	Client Satisfaction Survey	
Do you own a dog, cat or other pets?	Dogyesno	Catyesno
How many dogs/cats do you own?	Dog1 2 3 More: how many?	Cat1 2 3 More: how many?
Which dog/cat breeds are they?	Dog: _____	Cat:_____
How many other pets and which species?	Pets: Species:	
Are you a new or old customer?	New☐	Old☐
How often do you visit the Happy Veterinary Practice per year?	Only once☐ 1 – 3 x per year☐ 4 – 6x per year☐ More than 6 x per year☐	
What is your main reason for the visit?	Yearly vaccination☐ Health check up☐ Illness☐ Surgery☐ Grooming☐ Boarding☐ Buying pet food☐ Others, please specify☐	
How is the range of services and treatment?	Good☐Ok☐Poor☐	
How is the staff experience and skills?	Good☐Ok☐Poor☐	
Is the staff courteous and polite?	Good☐Ok☐Poor☐	
How are the facilities for out-patient treatment?	Good☐Ok☐Poor☐	
How are the facilities for in-patient treatment?	Good☐Ok☐Poor☐	
How are the treatment prices charged?	Good☐Ok☐Poor☐	
How are health packages charged?	Good☐Ok☐Poor☐	
How are emergencies handled?	Good☐Ok☐Poor☐	
How are the opening hours?	Good☐Ok☐Poor☐	
Is the waiting time reasonable?	Good☐Ok☐Poor☐	
Do you have suggestions for improvement?		

11.8.2. Survey Results and Interpretation

From the survey questionnaire, the final results can be grouped into information of the clients which will provide details about frequency of visits, animals in the client's household and visit reason and ratings that can be calculated to get the final results. For the standardized closed questions, a 3-point scale can be used to keep the questions simple and easy to answer. In the 3-point scale, 3 indicate good, 2 OK and 1 relates to poor on the attributes of veterinary practice services. This results in a maximum mean rating of 3.

Ratings can be grouped as follows:

After having calculated all mean results for the questions, the survey can establish the areas with high and low client satisfaction. All attributes falling under those areas can be put together in a table for comparison.

Table 11.3. Sample survey rating result for attribute range of services and treatment

Rating on range of service and treatment	% answered	% answered	% answered
	2009	2010	2011
Good	87.7	95.4	99.1
Ok	7.9	2.8	0
Poor	3.5	0	0.9
Not answered	0.9	3	0
Mean rating	2.85	2.89	2.98

Table 11.4. Areas of high client satisfaction

Attribute	2009	2010	2011
Range of services and treatments	2.85	2.89	2.98
Experience and skills of staff	2.90	2.92	2.97
Politeness of staff	2.89	2.89	2.95
Treatment charges	2.85	2.72	2.95
Health Care packages provided	2.89	2.83	2.94
Handling of any emergency situation	2.64	2.63	2.76
Opening hours are reasonable	1.93	2.20	2.41

Table 11.5. Areas of low client satisfaction

Attribute	2009	2010	2011
Facilities provided for out-patient treatment	1.41	1.62	1.98
Facilities provided for in-patient treatment	1.35	1.54	1.89
Waiting Time is reasonable	1.52	1.87	1.72

Apart from areas of high and low client satisfaction, it is also possible to have areas of significant variances for high and low satisfaction. This means that major jumps in ratings either up or down can be observed. High jumps in ratings reflect areas of significant variances for high satisfaction. Values with peaks followed by declines lead to significant variances for low client satisfaction.

The next step in the evaluation of the client satisfaction survey is the overall rating.

From those rating results, the conclusion can be drawn. Moreover, it becomes clearly visible which areas are areas of excellence, key strength areas and critical area for improvement. In the example above, the survey shows clear results that the Happy Veterinary Practice has major problems with its facilities, either for out-patients or in-patients.

This leads to the problems with workflow and thus resulting in longer waiting and low client satisfaction in this area. In such a case, a conclusion will definitely put the existing facilities into question as the other attributes like staff, service and pricing are positively received by the clients.

A recommendation in this case would be to review the practice facility's situation and to either look into areas of improvement through expansion of facilities or moving into new and better facilities.

Table 11.6. Overall rating of client satisfaction survey

Attribute	2009	2010	2011
Range of services and treatments	2.85	2.89	2.98
Experience and skills of staff	2.90	2.92	2.97
Politeness of staff	2.89	2.89	2.95
Treatment charges	2.85	2.72	2.95
Health Care packages provided	2.89	2.83	2.94
Handling of any emergency situation	2.64	2.63	2.76
Opening hours are reasonable	1.93	2.20	2.41
Facilities provided for out-patient treatment	1.41	1.62	1.98
Facilities provided for in-patient treatment	1.35	1.54	1.89
Waiting Time is reasonable	1.52	1.87	1.72
Average	2.32	2.31	2.55

After the conclusions, the survey needs to mention the action plan for corrective action, strengthening perceptions and recognition of excellent performance. It is highly important that the action plan will be reinforced by taking appropriate action that gets implemented. It is not the ideas of such a survey just to get beautiful data but not to use them for the improvement of the veterinary practice and hospital. Good attributes have to be strengthened to keep them on the high level in the coming year. Staff that works excellent has to be rewarded as a motivation tool. Rewards can be either in a monetary form but also in special training courses of advanced professional education or additional leave days.

11.9. CONCLUSION

Excellent client management is one of the key success factors for the profitable veterinary practice or hospital. A lot of factors influence the relationship between pet owners and the veterinary practice. This leads from the first phone call over the reception atmosphere to waiting time and finally interaction with the veterinary team and veterinary practitioner. In all these areas, problems and misunderstanding can arise. It is mandatory that the receptionist as well as the rest of the veterinary team work in the utmost polite way and try to create a friendly atmosphere for the pet owner. The client's first impression of the veterinary practice and hospital will lead to the famous "make it" or "break it". And if the practice does not "make it", a staggering 38% of pet owners will not return to the veterinary practice after their first visit, which will lead to a major loss of income. The secret to avoid this economic disaster for the veterinary practice is to offer attentive, personalized care for pet owners and to let them feel that everything possible is done for their beloved pet. This includes the right way of talking to them in a language they understand and that is not full of veterinary medical scientific terms. Care means to follow up with pet owners about the condition of the patients.

Complaints have to be dealt with in a professional way. They should be regarded by veterinary practitioners or practice managers not as a nuisance but as real help to identify problem areas. If no client would point out weak areas, the danger would be that possibly other clients will feel the same but not complain und subsequently leave the veterinary practice. However, complaining pet owners should not be mistaken with difficult clients. Three categories of difficult clients can be differentiated. They all require specific ways of handling them in the best way depending upon if they are difficult in the negative sense or just time consuming and therefore positively difficult. A positive perception of the reception staff can lead to a major reduction of so-called difficult clients as they are not difficult per se, but made difficult in the eye of the client.

An excellent way of understanding client behavior and satisfaction in a better way is the use of client satisfaction surveys. They are tremendously valuable to compare possible positive or negative changes in client satisfaction and their reason over a period of time. However, the idea of a client satisfaction survey is not just to have a nice survey to show off. The real value is to use the problem areas as basis for an action plan. The action plan may include improvement measures and even workflow changes if required. If implemented in a well structured way, pet owners can greatly benefit from improvement measures in the veterinary practice. A positive trend of increasing ratings in all survey areas should be observed over the years.

The benefit of all above mentioned measures is the increased satisfaction of clients resulting in improved compliance and therefore patients care as well as increased income and profit of veterinary practices and hospitals.

REFERENCES

[1]   AAHA. (2003). The path to high-quality care. Practical tips for improving compliance. *2002 AAHA Compliance study.* American Animal Hospital Association.

[2]   AAHA. (2009). Compliance. Taking quality care to the next level. Executive summary. *2008 AAHA Compliance study.* American Animal Hospital Association. http://www.aahanet.org/protected/ComplianceExecutivesummary0309.pdf   (Accessed on July 24th, 2011).

[3]   Ackermann, Lowell (2007). Blackwell's five-minute veterinary practice management consult. *Blackwell Publishing.* Iowa. USA.

[4]   Jevring, C. (2005). Compliance in veterinary practice.EJCAP. Vol. 15, issue 2; October, pp. 205-209.http://www.fecava.org/files/ejcap/281.pdf (Accessed on July 24th, 2011).

[5]   Shilcock, M. and Stutchfield, G.(2008). Veterinary practice management. *A practical guide.* Reprinted, Saunders, Elsevier Ltd. Philadelphia.

Chapter 12

OPERATIONS MANAGEMENT

ABSTRACT

Operations management is not a commonly used approach to veterinary practice routine. Coming from the business world, many veterinarians do not understand or underestimate the use of operations management procedures to speed up the practice's workflow. As the same operations management tools are applicable for veterinary work processes, this chapter takes the entirely new approach in veterinary practice management to explain in detail how to maximize work output by breaking down work processes into single stages. This helps to identify lost time, which can be tremendously reduced by realigning work processes and changing work layouts. Innovation and creativity are the keys in maximizing work processes to save valuable time for clients. This chapter will introduce the reader to a completely new and innovative mindset on how to look at veterinary work processes and layouts. Detailed step-by-step explanation will provide the reader with tools to adopt those measures in their daily practice routine in an easily understandable way.

12.1. INTRODUCTION

The choice of the veterinary services depends largely on the pet owner clientele of the veterinary practice. A very helpful tool in the evaluation of suitable services is a market study. A veterinary practice in a city area with mainly flats and high-rise building should concentrate more on services for feline patients than on canines as the number of cats will be most likely higher. The same applies to a very poor income area. Extraordinary services like very expensive surgeries might not be affordable for the clientele. However, the most important basic veterinary services should always be offered like vaccinations, neutering, small surgeries for injuries or minor disease and parasitoses. At the same time, a frequent client complaint is a too long waiting time. What can be done to reduce the waiting time without impacting the quality of care and efficiency of services? In order to speed up workflow and reduce waiting times, the work processes have to be designed in the most efficient way possible. This can be achieved by breaking down work processes into single work stages as this will help to cut out lost time. They can be rearranged in a more efficient way. Cycle calculations show considerable time differences before and after workflow process breakdown.

12.2. PROCESS DESIGN

For the service sector, a special service-process model exists, which integrates three different categories ranging from professional services, service shops to mass services [2].

High performance in jobs and their redesign is another vital driver of process design. Four different areas can contribute to improved job performance: span of control, span of accountability, span of influence and span of support. By widening or reducing any of these spans, a varied job output is the result thus enhancing the staff performance [6]. Furthermore the design of jobs includes three major areas for feasibility: technical, economic and behavior [2]. Moreover, the improved job design contributes to better productivity [3].

Benchmarking systems in hospitals are also useful in the resource planning and restructuring of patient-care processes [1].

In order to assess the process performance, several parameters have to be taken into consideration. One is to set up a detailed micro-process map [7], which breaks down all activities in the processes. Moreover, a precise step-by-step flow chart can help in finding out bottlenecks and to count the cycle time being the "average time between units of output emerging from the process" [7, p.109]. This will be explained in detail later in this chapter.

The layout of the position, process, cell and product is essential for the complete operation. However, sometimes a mixture of different layouts can be chosen according to the work type [7].

12.2.1. Existing Process Design

The right setting up of the service process design is another critical success factor of the veterinary practice. In order to evaluate the processes of the veterinary practices, the existing processes of the veterinary and laboratory work as well as the administration have to be carefully examined. The layout of the veterinary practices is usually a mixed layout with the following specifications [4]:

- Fixed-position layout: animals in the surgery room as they cannot be moved to another place
- Process layout: X-Ray, endoscopy unit, laboratory unit, hospitalization wards
- Cell layout: Intensive care unit

All processes have to be broken down and mapped in sub-steps. The veterinary team members being responsible for performing the individual processes need to be defined. This results in a set of maps, which are combined of veterinary medical process maps, laboratory process maps and administrative process maps [4].

When reviewing the processes, several bottlenecks in the veterinary work as well as laboratory work can normally be observed. This may include the reception which has a long waiting time thus sometimes leading to a reduced customer satisfaction. The same applies to the parasitological examination of fecal samples. Therefore, these two examples were chosen to be further reviewed in order to find ways for improvement.

12.2.2. Flow Process Chart

In order to assess the process performance, several parameters have to be taken into consideration like micro-process maps and workflow charts. At first, a flow process chart has been designed in order to show complete current process steps one after each other. This can be achieved by setting up a detailed micro-process map [7], which breaks down all activities in the processes. Moreover, a precise step-by-step flow chart can help in finding out potential bottlenecks.

The flow process chart requires correct time taking. This can be performed with a stop watching following an employee who performs a single procedure. The time stopped being then written down is used for the cycle time calculations. Although staff might be a little bit irritated when stopping their time they get used to it very easily. However, care needs to be taken that they perform their work in normal time and not speed up because they see the practice manager following them with the stop watch.

Special symbols are used to clarify activates in the flow process chart. They may contain operational activity, waiting time delays as well as deliberate storage which is neither waiting time nor a delay. The movement or transport as well as checking and examination are mapped, too.

Explanation of mapping symbols:

- Operational activity○
- Waiting time delay▢
- Deliberate storage (not waiting time or delay) ▽

- Movement, transport⇨
- Checking and examination▢

12.2.2.1. Flow Process Charts Examples

Example 1: Existing Registration Process for the Pet Owner in the Reception

As the first example, the waiting time problem at receptions will be reviewed as an example. This helps greatly in the evaluation of unnecessary waiting time for the clients, bottlenecks and areas where a restructuring of the process flow is urgently required. In 3 different examples, the detailed workflow charts are explained.

Example 2: Blood Examination

As the second example, we take the blood examination. In this example, we take the assumption that no hematology analyzer is available in the veterinary practice, and hematological samples have to be processed manually. The blood biochemistry is conducted by a fully automated biochemistry machine. Currently, one biochemistry machine exists in the laboratory. However, the biochemistry machine needs 2-3 minutes waiting time for calibration between two consecutive samples and 20 minutes to finish one processed sample. Moreover, the biochemistry machine needs frequent attention as often errors occur due to overheating or blood samples with very high values which the machine runs again [4].

At first, a flow process chart has to be designed for the blood examination in order to show complete current process steps one after each other. The blood examination consists of two parts: the hematological examination and the biochemical blood examination. Usually, one or maximum two laboratory technicians are performing this work.

Table 12.1. Sample flow process chart for veterinary practice:existing registration process for the pet owner in the reception [5]

S.No	Description of process step	Process flow	Time in Minutes
1	Pet owner arrives and goes to reception		0.30
2	Waiting at reception until receptionist serves pet owner		5.00
3	Receptionist takes owner and pet's information		1.00
4	Receptionist enters data in software and searches patient file		1.00
5	File found, receptionist asks for reason of visit		0.30
6	Owner explains visit reason		3.00
7	Receptionist asks pet owner to wait for the consultation		0.30
8	Pet owner sits down and waits for consultation		15.00
	Total time		25.90

The result shows that one single hematological blood examination takes 17.26 minutes and the biochemistry 30.10 minutes if there are no machine problems.

The machine layout in the blood laboratory is shown below.

Example 3: Parasitological Feces Examination

Another frequent test in the veterinary practice is the parasitological examination of feces for parasites or bacteria. The animal's feces is either given by the owner to the receptionist in the reception or taken in the examination room by the veterinary technician.

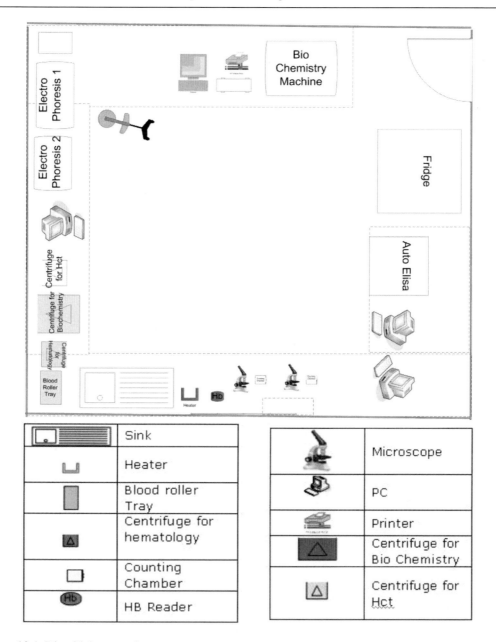

Figure 12.1. Blood laboratory layout.

12.2.2.2. Flow Process Breakdown of Walking Time

The walking time of veterinary staff needs to be calculated that is required to conduct daily work processes. This includes the distance that is traveled one way as well as the per diem distance traveled. Then the walking time in second or minutes between different locations has to be assessed.

For simplification purposes, we assume that all three examples happen in a large veterinary practice or hospital. The location of the parasitology laboratory is at the other end of the practice building in the laboratory area.

Table 12.2. Sample flow process chart for veterinary practice:
Existing flow process chart for blood examination [4]

S.No	Description of process step	Process flow	Time in Minutes
1	Taking blood from roller tray and putting BC tube in centrifuge		0.15
2	Putting blood for hematology in Hb test machine		0.17
3	Dilution of blood for WBC count		1.10
4	Dilution of blood for RBC count		0.39
5	Finishing of Hb test		0.29
6	Preparation of blood smear and putting for drying		0.19
7	Reading Hb test and writing result in book		0.35
8	Preparation of Hct test and putting in centrifuge		0.57
9	Staining of blood smear		1.19
10	Waiting time		0.19
11	Centrifugation of BC blood finished		0.45
12	Preparation of BC blood for machine and entering data in PC		0.07
13	Loading BC machine		0.45
14	Waiting time		0.56
15	Start of WBC and RBC count		3.12
16	Finished WBC RBC count		0.23
17	Opening of Hct centrifuge		0.17
18	Hct count		0.19
19	Start to check stained smear slide under microscope		4.34
20	Finished check of smear slide and Writing result in book		0.23
21	Waiting time until BC machine finished		11.44
	Total time		30.10

Table 12.3. Sample flow process chart for veterinary practice: existing flow process chart for parasitological feces examination [4]

S.No	Description of process step	Process flow	Time in Minutes
1	Preparation and mixing of fecal for direct smear test		1.09
2	Microscopic examination		3.01
3	Result writing		0.32
4	Flotation preparation		1.22
5	Waiting time till flotation is settled		4.58
6	Preparing slide of flotation		0.01
7	Microscopic examination		0.45
8	Result writing		0.30
	Total time		12.18

The distances between the reception are respective examination room to the parasitology laboratory is 56 meter respectively 55 meter. Therefore, the walking time between the different rooms needs to be taken into consideration. First, it is necessary to count the times the distance is traveled one-way [4]. This can be shown in a table.

Table 12.4. Daily distance traveled one way [4]

To \ From	Reception	Examination room	Blood laboratory	Parasitology laboratory
Reception	---	150	---	25
Examination room	120	---	65	85
Blood laboratory	---	45	---	20
Parasitology laboratory	20	85	60	---

As next step, the daily distance traveled has to be calculated in a table.

Table 12.5. Daily distance traveled [4]

To \ From	Reception	Examination room	Blood laboratory	Parasitology laboratory
Reception	---	270	---	45
Examination room		---	110	170
Blood laboratory			---	80
Parasitology laboratory				---

The next step is the calculation of the walking time between the different rooms. The walking time from reception to the blood or parasitology laboratory takes 1.02 minutes. The travel time between the examination room and the blood or parasitology laboratory is 0.51 minutes. The time distance between the reception and examination room is 0.05 minutes and between the blood and parasitology laboratory is 0.08 minutes. With regard to the number of times certain ways are walked, the time traveled in minutes per distance daily is as follows:

Table 12.6. Daily walking time [4]

Distance between	Number of walks	Distance in minutes	Daily time in minutes
reception to examination room	270	0.08	22.00
reception to parasitology laboratory	45	1.02	46.30
examination room to blood laboratory	110	1.02	112.20
examination room to parasitology laboratory	170	0.51	87.10
blood laboratory to parasitology laboratory	80	0.08	6.40

12.2.3. Cycle Time

The next step following the evaluation of the workflow is the identification of the cycle time. The counting of the cycle time being the "average time between units of output emerging from the process" [7, p.109] is another helpful tool in improving the workflow.

It is important to calculate the cycle time required in order to assess the stages of individual processes [7].

The cycle time can be defined as [7]:

$$\textbf{Cycle time for the layout} = \frac{\textbf{time available}}{\textbf{number of registrations}}$$

Example 1: Existing Registration Process for the Pet Owner in the Reception [5]

Now we return to our workflow example at the reception. Regarding the registration of visits in a veterinary practice, in the peak time 30 pets are visiting the practice per day (150 vaccinations per week) and the time available for registrations is 40 hours per week [4]. The cycle time for the reception can be calculated as follows:

$$\text{Cycle time for the layout} = \frac{\text{time available}}{\text{number of registrations}}$$

$$= \frac{40 \text{ hours}}{150 \text{ (vaccinations)}} = \frac{40 \times 60 \text{ minutes}}{150} = 16 \text{ minutes}$$

This means that a maximum of 16 minutes per registration should be allowed.

To improve and speed up the work process, it is essential to get the number of work stages. Therefore, the total work content has to be calculated [7]. The maximum time for the registration of a pet owner in the reception is 25.90 minutes in our workflow chart example above.

$$\text{Number of stages} = \frac{\text{total work content}}{\text{required cycle time}}$$

$$= \frac{25.90 \text{ minutes}}{16 \text{ minutes}}$$

$$= \underline{1.6 \text{ stages or rounded up 2 stages}}$$

Blood Examination

Regarding the previous examples of blood examination, in the peak time 45 blood samples are examined per day (225 samples per week) and the time available for examination is 40 hours per week [4].

The cycle time can be calculated as follows:

$$\text{Cycle time for the layout} = \frac{\text{time available}}{\text{Number of samples to be processed}}$$

$$= \frac{40 \text{ (hours)}}{225 \text{ (samples)}} = \frac{40\times60 \text{ minutes}}{225} = \underline{11.07 \text{ minutes}}$$

To improve and speed up the process of the blood diagnostic, it is essential to get the number of stages. Therefore, the total work content has to be calculated [7]. The maximum time for the biochemical blood examination is 30.10 minutes and for the hematological examination 17.26 minutes.

Blood biochemistry examination:

$$\text{Number of stages} = \frac{\text{total work content for biochemistry}}{\text{required cycle time}}$$

$$= \frac{30.10 \text{ minutes}}{11.06 \text{ minutes}}$$

$$= \underline{2.72 \text{ stages or rounded up 3 stages}}$$

Blood hematology examination:

$$\text{Number of stages} = \frac{\text{total work content for hematology}}{\text{required cycle time}}$$

$$= \frac{17.26 \text{ minutes}}{11.06 \text{ minutes}}$$

$$= \underline{1.56 \text{ stages or rounded up 2 stages}}$$

Parasitological Feces Examination

Regarding the previous examples of blood examination, in the peak time 85 feces samples are examined per day (425 samples per week) and the time available for examination is 40 hours per week [4].

The cycle time can be calculated as follows [7]:

$$\text{Cycle time for the layout} = \frac{\text{time available}}{\text{Number of samples to be processed}}$$

$$= \frac{40 \ (hours)}{425 \ (samples)} = \frac{40 \times 60 \ \ minutes}{425} = 6.05 \ minutes$$

To shorten the parasitological examination time, again the number of stages and the total work content has to be calculated [7]. The maximum time for the direct smear fecal examination is 4.42 minutes and for the complete parasitological examination including flotation 12.18 minutes.

Direct smear examination:

$$\text{Number of stages} = \frac{\text{total work content for direct smear}}{\text{required cycle time}}$$

$$= \frac{4.42 \ minutes}{6.05 \ minutes}$$

$$= 0.73 \ \text{stages or rounded up 1 stage}$$

Flotation examination:

$$\text{Number of stages} = \frac{\text{total work content for flotation}}{\text{required cycle time}}$$

$$= \frac{12.18 \ minutes}{6.05 \ minutes}$$

12.3. IMPROVED PROCESS AND PRODUCT DESIGNS

The setting up of detailed workflow charts and cycle times shed light on potential problem areas and lost time. The next step is the redesign of the process maps. This includes the changes in practice and room layouts as well work flows. Limitations in building constructions or number of staff might sometimes lead to compromises between desired process change and automation and the possible process change.

12.3.1. Layout Change

Layout changes include changes to the existing set-up of equipments and machineries by rearranging them in a way that follows the workflow. They might also contain structural changes like shifting equipment in another room to save walking time. Hereby hygienic considerations and building design need to be considered. In our examples, the redesign of the process maps have to consider the hygienic conditions in the laboratory and the available laboratory staff being currently four laboratory technicians. For example 1, the waiting area and examination room's layout cannot be changed due to building design restrictions. In the second example, the blood laboratory cannot be relocated due to the hygiene and safety reasons. However, the fact that in the third example a large amount of time gets lost while walking between the examination room to the parasitology laboratory leads to the conclusion that the layout of the parasitology laboratory should be changed.

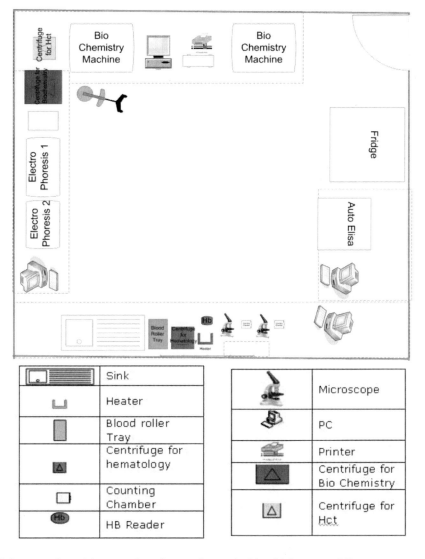

Figure 12.2. Improved machinery and equipment layout in blood laboratory [4].

Example 1: Registration Process for the Pet Owner in the Reception

No layout change can be done.

Example 2: Blood Examination

Due to hygiene and safety reasons, the blood laboratory has to be located further away from the clinical area although this increases the walking time to the laboratory. However, the work can be split among three laboratory technicians by simple relocating of some of the machines and equipment inside the blood laboratory. An additional new second biochemistry machine should be integrated in the laboratory layout and workflow. Machines and equipment have been relocated according to work areas like biochemistry and hematology.

Example 3: Parasitological Feces Examination

A layout change for parasitology laboratory cannot be performed, but another solution can be found to save walking time. One possibility is to keep a microscope with one laboratory technician in the examination room which can be done without hygienic concerns. This results in a distance of 0.17 minutes from reception to the newly designated parasitology area and from examination room to this place of 0.11 minutes. The total time saved through this layout change is 38.25 minutes per day from the reception and 68 minutes from the examination room to the new parasitology area.

12.3.2. Workflow Change

The workflow changes are introduced according to the results in the cycle time and walking time calculation. Workflow changes also depend on the number of staff and their professional abilities. In order to improve the processes, the number of stages in which the process needs to be broken down have to re revisited and revised. The number of stages has been already calculated in our examples.

Example 1: Registration Process for the Pet Owner in the Reception

The result of this example is that the registration time has to be rearranged and split in two stages, e.g. in a sole registering of owner and patient at the reception and then transfer of the pet owner into a special room for taking the information for the practice visit by a qualified veterinary nurse who asks for the case history and already prepares e.g. the vaccination for the veterinarian. This will lead not only to a reduced waiting time for the client but also to a reduced treatment time for the veterinarian as well.

Example 2: Blood Examination

As time is lost through waiting and unequal distribution of workflow, the work needs to be balanced and equally distributed. Moreover, one additional biochemistry machine is required to speed up the process and run more samples at a time. Furthermore, it will serve as a backup machine in case of technical failure of one machine. Therefore, the investment of purchasing a new biochemistry machine is justified and economically valid. However, it is impossible to break the biochemistry work in 3 stages. By dividing the time between 2 machines can double the quantities of samples to be run and working on the Hct count. This workflow can be regarded as a 3 stage work, too.

Table 12.7. Balanced workflow for blood examination: Biochemistry [4]

S.No	Description of process step	Process flow	Time in Minutes
1	Taking blood from roller tray and putting BC tube in centrifuge		0.15
2	Preparation of Hct test and putting in centrifuge		0.57
3	Centrifugation of BC blood finished		1.11
4	Preparation of BC blood for machine and entering data in PC		0.07
5	Loading BC machine		0.45
6	Opening of Hct centrifuge		0.17
7	Hct count		0.19
	Total time		3.11

The hematology work has been spilt in 2 parts for 2 technicians, one for WBC and RBC count as well as Hb test and the second one for the examination of the blood smear. The calculated 2 stages can be achieved in this way.

Table 12.8. Balanced workflow for blood examination: WBC, RBC count and Hb [4]

S.No	Description of process step	Process flow	Time in Minutes
2	Putting blood for hematology in Hb test machine		0.17
3	Dilution of blood for WBC count		1.10
4	Dilution of blood for RBC count		0.39
5	Finishing of Hb test		0.29
7	Reading Hb test and writing result in book		0.35
15	Start of WBC and RBC count		3.12
16	Finished WBC RBC count and result writing		0.23
	Total time		6.05

The procedure should be as follows: while one slide is drying, another already dried slide can be stained and checked under the microscope. After this is resulted and the result is written, a new slide can be prepared and put for drying. The previously done slide has finished drying in the meantime and can go for staining and checking. This means that always at least 2 slides will be done on a rotation basis in order to avoid waiting time for the drying process.

Table 12.9. Balanced workflow for blood examination: blood smear [4]

S.No	Description of process step	Process flow	Time in Minutes
6	Preparation of blood smear and putting for drying		0.19
9	Staining of blood smear		1.19
19	Check stained smear slide under microscope		4.34
20	Finished check of smear slide and result writing		0.23
	Total time		6.35

Table 12.10. Balanced workflow for parasitological fecal examination [4]

S.No	Description of process step	Process flow	Time in Minutes
1	Flotation preparation		1.22
2	Preparation and mixing of fecal for direct smear test		1.09
3	Microscopic examination		3.01
4	Result writing		0.32
5	Waiting time till flotation is finished		0.16
6	Preparing slide of flotation		0.01
7	Microscopic examination		0.45
8	Result writing		0.30
	Total time		6.56

Example 3: Parasitological Feces Examination

As time is lost through walking long distances and waiting time for the flotation examination, the work needs to be balanced and equally distributed. The number of calculated stages for the direct smear method is 1 stage, which is matching with the balanced workflow. The flotation was calculated to have 2 stages, which are integrated in the new workflow by starting the complete fecal examination process with the flotation preparation. Then the direct smear method will be performed in the waiting time until the flotation is settled. The only waiting time is now reduced to 0.16 minutes from the previous 4.58 minutes until the flotation is settled, which cannot be done in a different way as this is the time required. This leads to a much faster and more efficient fecal examination while avoiding unnecessary waiting times.

Therefore, the calculated cycle time is 6.05 minutes, which is almost fulfilled with the rearranged workflow with 6.56 minutes being due to the required waiting and examination time.

12.4. STANDARDIZATION OF SERVICES

Standardization is defined as "the degree to which processes, products or services are prevented from varying over time" [7, p.778]. This leads to a restricted variety of services to an extent that the real value for the client can be achieved. Standardized services have common elements within the "package" which can be regarded as sub-components. Therefore, these sub-components are interchangeable and can be used for services and processes in different ways [7]. This does not mean that services cannot be performed according to the requirements of the individual patient, but that they follow a clearly defined and fewer varied path. This can be applied for example to special consultations like pediatric or geriatric examinations, which can integrate several pre-defined steps. Such pre-defined steps can be entered in the internal policies and procedures of the veterinary practice. This enables new staff members or even existing employees to review those procedures and perform them in the same way. The advantage is that new employees adapt much faster to the way how procedures are performed in the veterinary practice which saves considerable time and reduces mistakes. Moreover, it ensures that all team members follow the same routine which creates an improved control over performed work processes with enhanced patient care.

12.5. CONCLUSION

Operations management is often not the favorite subject for veterinary practitioners and veterinary personnel. Often it is regarded as difficult and only usable for manufacturing companies. However, the opposite is the case: operations management rightly adopted in the veterinary practice can save considerable time and tremendously improve service quality and subsequent patient care. To integrate main principles in the daily practice routine the existing work processes in all practice departments have to be reviewed and assessed. This can be done in the very practical way of using a stop watch to measure the time employees need to perform individual work processes. The single process micro steps and their respective time are then entered in the work process chart. This helps to understand where time is really lost and where a real deliberate waiting time, e.g. for processing a consultation or laboratory sample exists. Movements of staff as well as transport time for animals or samples are assessed and entered in daily walking charts. The calculation of the cycle time leads to very interesting results on how many stages a process entails. These data build the baseline for improved process and products designs. Changes in the practice or room layout have to be considered to reduce walking time or to put equipments together in a way that the complete work process can be performed in one place. The workflow changes come as the final step. After revisiting the number of process stages, workflow changes include the rearrangement of staff, adjustments in procedures or even investment in new equipments. However, some parameters cannot be changed due to external circumstances like practice building construction. In such cases, a compromise between desired process change and the possible process change needs to be found. If used correctly, veterinary practices can benefit greatly from the integration of operations management in their daily practice routine with satisfied clients as the reward.

REFERENCES

[1]   Linna, M. (2006). Benchmarking hospital productivity. Health Policy Monitor. Survey.No.7.http://www.healthpolicymonitor.org/en/About_Us/Partner_Institutions/ST AKES/Benchmarking_hospital_productivity.html(Accessed on June 24th, 2006).

[2]   McMillan, R. and Mullen, T. (2005a). *Operations management.* Volume 1. 3rd ed. Glasgow: The Graduate School of Business University of Strathclyde.

[3]   McMillan, R. and Mullen, T. (2005b). *Operations management.* Volume 2. 3rd ed. Glasgow: The Graduate School of Business University of Strathclyde.

[4]   Muller, M.G. and Abu Aabed, A. (2006). *Operations management.* MBA Assignment.University of Strathclyde. Graduate School of Business. Glasgow, UK.

[5]   Müller, M.G. and Abu Aabed, A. (2007). Guidelines for setting up a small and medium size enterprise. MBA Thesis, University of Strathclyde. Graduate School of Business. Glasgow, UK.

[6]   Simons, R. (2005). Designing high performance jobs. *Harvard Business Review.* July-August. pp. 55-62.

[7]   Slack, N., Chambers, S. and Johnston, R. (2004). *Operations management.* 4th ed. Prentice Hall. Financial Times.

Chapter 13

SUPPLY CHAIN MANAGEMENT, OUTSOURCING AND INVENTORY

ABSTRACT

Supply-chain management has recently undergone a lot of changes in recent times. This chapter introduces the different ways of supply-chain management and their meaning for the veterinary practice. Moreover, a relatively new feature in the veterinary practice management is outsourcing. Outsourcing has many advantages but also disadvantages.

This chapter highlights the positive use of outsourcing, but critically reflects on its negative impacts for veterinary practices and hospitals. In this context, the highly important issue of stock control and inventory gets discussed. Inventory is a very critical part of veterinary practice management but is often underestimated and not processed in the right way.

It includes not only medicines, but machinery and equipments, too. Stock control is required to keep track on stock movement. It is inevitable to reduce stock losses and wrong ordering practices. Stock movement needs to be analyzed to understand better opportunities of additional income through fast moving items.

13.1. INTRODUCTION

The ordering process, supply-chain management, stock control and inventory play an important part in the veterinary practice management. They do not only help in securing sufficient supplies for the smooth running of the practice but also provide adequate inventory stocks according to the individual needs and requirements of the veterinary practice.

Medicine and consumables stocks can be controlled very well through proper supply-chain management and inventory control as this will reduce the number of expired items and prevent lack of required medicines. But what does supply-chain management really mean?

13.2. SUPPLY-CHAIN MANAGEMENT (SCM) AND THE INCREASING ROLE OF E-BUSINESS PRACTICES

13.2.1. Definition and SCM Parts

Supply chain is defined as "the flow of materials, information, money, and services from raw materials suppliers through factories and warehouses to the end customers" [19, p.48] which means in our case the veterinary practice. Moreover, the supply chain is divided into three parts being upstream, internal and downstream. Upstream processes involve mainly suppliers whereas internal processes include the in-house processes. On the other hand, downstream supply chain is the end of the chain, the delivery of goods and services to the end customer and consumers [19]. The SCM is closely related with the value chain that provides information about the value added to the company. Therefore, e-commerce and e-business add value to the company and the SCM through new business models and automated business processes and restructuring of outdated processes [14, 19]. This applies in the same way to veterinary practices.

In the supply-chain management, several developments are currently under processing like cost cutting of supplies and procurement and reduced inventory costs. Moreover, timely deliveries become more important as well as quality control and product specifications. Larger powerful manufacturers try to get more power and influence on their suppliers where in the same time the distribution of many smaller suppliers is another new development [8, 14].

13.2.2. SCM Infomediaries

The traditional intermediaries in the SCM are brokers who provide services for sellers and buyers. However, intermediaries can be found in the e-business, too. These so-called infomediaries are also used to control the massive information flows, consolidate the information and then sell them to customers. The infomediaries hold an important position in the e-world because they provide services that might be unfeasible for customers. They also bridge the gap of limitation for producers and consumers like search costs, lack of privacy or incomplete information if the customer requests more information than provided by the seller. Moreover, as some customers do not want to pay, infomediaries are used to minimize the contract risk. They also help in negotiations for pricing inefficiencies between manufacturers and consumers. In supply-chain management, B2B infomediaries have found their way into e-business as the so-called e-distributors [14, 19].

13.2.3. Supply-Chain Management and Changes through E-Business

E-business provides an extended area of opportunities for the supply-chain management. These opportunities lie in purchasing requirements, potential supplier identification, deliverables negotiations and transactions completion. Another major part is the receiving, holding and location of supplies as well as monitoring of relationships and long-term value evaluation. E-procurement is another field of potential opportunities in the supply-chain management with the main focus on B2B relationships [8, 14].

Through e-business, the supply chain got transformed with major improvements like the hub-based chain. The electronic hub has become the center for all SCM activities using web-based enterprise resource planning systems like from SAP. These systems speed up orders and production cycle time immensely. This helps especially on a global range with designers, manufacturers or engineers located in other countries. It paves the way to virtual manufacturing where various manufacturing plants can be controlled and run by a single company, as if they were placed in the same location thus creating more transparency for the customers. Moreover, the previously paper-based ordering or invoicing has changed to B2B application performed online consequently creating a competitive advantage for the company [14, 19].

New features are mobile computing solutions, which are used to protect disruptions of the supply chain and for integration of business processes into the supply chain. These issues are emerging more and more in the wireless B2B world in which the collaboration among different supply chain partners gets more importance [14, 19].

13.2.4. Order Fulfillment and E-Business

The order fulfillment process has changed through the introduction of e-business, too. Online sales have to face with new pressuring issues like product line expansion and the delivery of large numbers of small product quantities. Moreover, customer expectations are growing more and more thus making order fulfillment more difficult [17]. After the order has been placed, the company needs to ensure the payment by the customer as otherwise the order will be delayed. After this initial control, the inventory needs to be checked if the ordered item or its components are available. Often direct connection between the order process and the inventory availability is done through integrated software programs. Once the availability of the product is confirmed, it will be shipped out as an insured item, if required [14, 19].

The main problem in order fulfillment is uncertainties, which are not fulfilling the forecasted demand of customers. This might be due to changed consumer behavior or technological innovations. Moreover, delayed delivery times as well as quality problems might seriously affect the order fulfillment. Other problems are the poor or lacking coordination of activities along the supply chain as well as the outsourced third party logistics which might be unreliable, delayed or not well coordinated. This affects mainly pure e-supply chains. The so-called bullwhip effect has a negative impact on an order which comes from traditional and e-supply chain in the same time. Hereby, the fluctuation of order might be so large that the forecasted demand cannot be met and thus firing back in many parts of the supply chain like inventory, shipping and order fulfillment [14, 19].

The above-mentioned problems can be solved through web-based ordering systems with enhanced accuracy. Moreover, e-marketplaces have eased those fulfillment problems as well as specialized warehouse inventory management solutions. Inventories in warehouses can be automated with specialized software for order taking and pick-up robots. Bar codes are identified at scanning stations and then send to their final destination [19]. Nowadays, the bar codes are in the process of being replaced by radio-frequency identification tags (RIDF) which use wireless technology, are programmable and can be used as tracking devices [8, 14].

13.2.5. Supply-Chain Management in Veterinary Practices

In veterinary medicine, large wholesale companies have entered the market with online shops and provide 24 hours ordering of medicines as well as consumables in many countries nowadays. This greatly helps to reduce large stocks of medicines, especially rarely used or very expensive ones, and consumables. Reduction of inventory costs and cost cutting of supplies is a very effective way to save expenses in the veterinary practice. This online ordering of medicines is exceedingly useful in the case of very special and rarely used medicines that are prescribed to a selected pet with this condition. Moreover, medicines with short expiry dates can be stocked to a minimum and therefore, do not have to be discarded unused after they expire.

It is advisable to have a selection of excellent veterinary wholesale companies which are providing 24 hours delivery services. As registered customer, veterinary practices will not only get the items in an easy and fast way, but they will also get notified from upcoming promotions and special sales. This can save a considerable amount of money.

13.3. INVENTORY AND STOCK MANAGEMENT IN VETERINARY PRACTICE

13.3.1. Inventory

Stock management and inventory are critical in the veterinary practice as the quality of medicines and their correct storage has to be controlled well to use them in the best way for the patients. However, stock management does not only include medicines, but also medical and laboratory consumables, and all items that are used in the veterinary practice. They can be instruments, machines and other equipments. Machines and computer hardware should be labeled preferably with a bar code. This will help to determine which equipment is stored in which room.

This labeling helps to control what is available but also to perform the annual inventory and asset management. A list that states all equipments per room is very valuable in performing an accurate and fast inventory. The fixed asset list does not only provide information about existing machinery and equipment but are required to assess the depreciation of individual items and to keep them up to date.

The pharmacy room should be located in a central, clean, dark and cool room in the veterinary practice. It must include a special safety cabinet for anesthetics or controlled drugs that can be locked with a key. All items have to be stored there, and the room needs to be locked at all times. Some medicines and especially vaccines have to be stored by 2-8°C in the refrigerator.

All items in the pharmacy or store have to be thoroughly recorded to avoid problems later. Special recording of controlled drugs is mandatory. It is also advisable to appoint one staff member as responsible staff for pharmacy and stock control. Nowadays, in most veterinary practice software, inventory modules are included. This has the major advantage that it is easier and more precise to control the stock of medicines, consumables and pet food. Usually, those inventory modules have all information about items such as:

- Item name
- Item batch number
- Item ID code or barcode
- Quantity
- Expiry date
- Reorder level/quantity
- Supplier name
- Supplier address
- Statistical information and reports

Optional features include:

- Automatic reorder from supplier when reaching reorder level
- Authorization for responsible staff
- Barcode reader

It is useful to dispense medicines and consumables weekly from the pharmacy as this leads to enhanced stock control and does not waste time by always going to get items from the pharmacy. Staff of different departments like consultation, surgery or radiology can request the required items from the responsible person who issues them from the pharmacy and changes their numbers automatically in the inventory.

When you buy an existing veterinary practice, you might already have some medicines that come with it. In such cases, it is necessary to establish a beginning quantity that states the previous stock. This beginning quantity can also reflect the stock at the beginning of the year. Then you get a received quantity which reflects the amount of ordered medicines. The issued quantity contains those medicines that have been dispensed to the different departments upon their request. The quantity that is left in the pharmacy is the quantity at hand. Remarks like store item in a fridge can be very helpful, especially when the originally appointed pharmacy responsible goes on leave, and another staff member takes over temporarily.

Table 13.1. Sample pharmacy stock details

Item name	Package	Unit	Expiry date	Beginning quantity	Received quantity	Issued quantity	Quantity on hand	Remarks
A	1 x 50	Bottle/ml	Jan 14	0	2	1	1	Store in fridge
B	1 x 30	Pack/tabl	Nov 13	0	10	2	8	
C	1 x 6	Pack/ pcs	Apr 14	2	5	3	4	
D	1 x 5	Amp/ml	Jun 13	0	25	5	20	
E	1 x 40	Tube/ g	Dec 15	4	0	2	2	
F	1 x 5	Tube/ml	Oct 14	0	50	22	28	

It is very useful to maintain a stock inventory of received items on a monthly basis. This help to track supplier deliveries.

Table 13.2. Sample pharmacy received stock details monthly

Item name	Package	Unit	Expiry date	Received quantity	Received from	Received on	Remarks
A	1 x 50	Bottle	Jan 14	10	Supplier 1	01/12/2011	Store in fridge
B	1 x 30	Pack	Nov 13	25	Supplier 2	05/12/2011	
C	1 x 6	Pack	Apr 14	40	Supplier 2	22/12/2011	
D	1 x 5	Amp	Jun 13	4	Supplier 3	08/12/2011	
E	1 x 40	Tube	Dec 15	12	Supplier 1	18/12/2011	
F	1 x 5	Tube	Oct 14	36	Supplier 3	23/12/2011	

The inventory of pharmacy items and equipments like fixed asserts is taken on a yearly basis. It should also be taken when the responsible staff is e.g. going on leave or cannot continue his function. Before the stock control goes over to another staff, a full inventory has to be taken, recorded and signed off by the old and new responsible staff.

The annual inventory and stock audit includes the current stock taking. The audit results are then compared with the stock taking at the beginning of the year. The purchased items are added to the beginning stock and the sold medicines, and items are deducted. This calculation has to provide the stock at the time of stock taking.

13.3.2. Stock Management

Stock, especially of medicines can be a very expensive part of the veterinary practice's budget. Therefore, it is vital that this stock is properly managed to avoid financial losses. Losses can occur due to expiry of items, uncorrected storage, damage to the packing units and their content and theft. Good pharmacy stock software will help to minimize such losses as it can remind the stock keeper of threatening expiry dates and reorder levels. Reorder levels of medicines and consumables help to reduce the amount of items carried in stock and thus reduce potential losses. This can be performed manually, too, but requires much more work and accurate entries in the stock keeping book. Good stock keeping also helps to reduce the risk of theft as all staff members know very well that the stock is fully under control, and every missing item will be detected easily. For this reason, it is mandatory to have one designated staff responsible of the pharmacy and stock because this reduces accessibility for other staff members drastically. Good and spacious storage facilities prevent damage to medicines and other items as they can be stored in shelves in a proper way without being crowded and pushed together.

Stock analysis is highly important to understand the stock movement and to avoid overstocking. Most important stock items can be analyzed according to the 80/20 rule. This means that 20% of stock items cause 80% of stock costs thus reflecting the 20% top selling products of the practice [18]. Those 20% top selling products should be analyzed very well as they can produce considerable income for the practice and have a major impact on stock movement.

Stock movement can be differentiated into sold items and used items. Sales of medicines and other products can greatly increase the income of the veterinary practice. They can be analyzed on a monthly basis. Used items are going out of the stock but are used, e.g. for hospitalized patients or during surgeries and treatment.

As stock can be considered as bound money, it is better to keep the stock as low as possible and to work with reorder levels. In some cases, it might be good to take offered discounts of wholesalers to save money, especially on fast moving items. Nevertheless, it should be calculated what approximate amount of items will be used to avoid overstocking. However, it does not make much sense to purchase large quantities of slow moving medicines or more stock that can be used in one year. Even the best discount does not help if the items' expiry and the invested money will be completely lost.

Although every veterinary pharmacy and stock have to contain all important medicines and products, it might be impossible to have all items on stock. Nowadays, very good wholesalers exist that can deliver medicines and product within 24 hours after ordering. This might be very useful in cases of rarely used medicines. Moreover, those companies offer to send the order without extra charges if a certain order level is exceeded. This can save a tremendous amount of time and money. In addition, it helps to reduce large stock quantities and expired items. These wholesalers offer discounted products and have sales for their loyal customers. It is therefore worth selecting one, two or three good wholesalers and to stick with them for orders.

13.4. Outsourcing

Outsourcing has become a global mega trend in different areas like information management, communications [3] and operations and administration management [4]. The main intention was originally to save costs [2]. Today, the big companies start outsourcing "core operations to third-party specialists in order to improve operational performance" [2, p.1]. Most outsourcing companies believe that outsourcing is based on partnerships and strategic alliances between company and vendor [7, 13]. However, this attitude has been criticized as the goals of the outsourcing company and the vendors are certainly different [1, 10]. A new emerging trend in the outsourcing world is offshore outsourcing to overseas countries. This volume has increased by 40% in 2003 and is likely to continue in the future [15]. Outsourcing has become the big global hype of our modern times. However, it needs to be carefully reviewed which departments or parts of a company are suitable for outsourcing. In fact, some companies are outsourcing their complete business nowadays. It is advisable that the core business should not be given to outsourcing vendors because otherwise the competitive advantage towards other competitors might get lost [5, 11]. The possible advantages and disadvantages or risks have to be carefully evaluated [1, 12].

13.4.1. Advantages

Outsourcing can help companies to get access to specialized and not yet available skills [5] and therefore to improve the quality [3]. Through outsourcing, access to better quality competencies and knowledge can be gained [9, 12]. Cost savings are beneficial especially for smaller companies due to economies of scale. Another important advantage is time savings and discovery of hidden costs. Outsourcing can be used also to concentrate more on the business core parts than to get entangled in a lot of outside activities [3]. Outsourcing can equally important provide a bigger flexibility in moving staff to other positions through in-house staff being free. Management has the possibility to concentrate better on its core business and improve the general productivity. Moreover, a good point for outsourcing is a better accountability of the vendor company [1, 3].

13.4.2. Disadvantages

A lot of people and companies believe that the outsourcing company and the vendor enter a partnership relation. This is not true as both parties have their own objectives and profit expectations [5]. A lot of outsourcing relationships are not really going smooth and well [5]. Despite the outsourcing boom, control of the business is lost to the vendor [3], but control is an often neglected topic [5]. It is almost impossible to reverse outsourcing [3] due to the loss of the company's own infrastructure and specialist staff [1, 5].

Another issue is costs that might increase after the initial stage. It does not happen in all outsourcing cases that the quality really improves. The capacity of the vendor might not be sufficient because vendors have multiple clients and do not give priority to one customer [3]. Through outsourcing, flexibility gets lost [3]. Only few outsourcing companies request performance measures of the vendor company which is usually stated in the contract. Moreover, it is not known if the outsourcing vendor shares the processing facilities with other outsourcing companies. This might include other potential business competitors [1, 5].

13.4.3. Outsourcing in Veterinary Practices

Outsourcing in the veterinary practice is a fairly new phenomenon that just started a few years back but has not reached the extent that outsourcing reaches in other branches. Why is outsourcing still not very much adopted in the veterinary practice business model? The main reason is the fact that veterinary practitioners prefer to keep all business parts in their own hand and not to look outside for other opportunities. It has been stated that veterinarians who do not venture quickly into outsourcing might suffer great disadvantages compared to their colleagues [6]. But is this really true?

At first, we can look at areas of the veterinary practice where outsourcing would be possible. This is mainly the administrative part, including accounting, financial planning, payroll processing, website, client communication and marketing [6]. Moreover, recruitment has been recommended as veterinary outsourcing [6]. When looking at those issues, it becomes clear that several factors determine a need for outsourcing. The main one is the qualification of staff for certain areas as well as the size of the veterinary practice or hospital. In a small one or two veterinarian practice, a lot of things can be performed in-house if the work volume is not exceeding an average workload. The external services of a certified public accountant [6] can help to bridge the gap between professional accounting work and no recruitment of an accountant in the veterinary practice. However, once the work volume exceeds the average workload or a larger size of the veterinary practice is reached, an administrator with accounting knowledge should be employed to ensure full financial control over income, expenses, cash flow and other financial statements. This might be more cost-effective than using an external certified public accountant in such a case as the accountant will have full-time work, and he can be used to help in another administrative work if he is willing to and able to multitask.

With regard to the website development, it is definitely advisable to use the services of a professional website design company. A professional website matching the corporate identity is a must for a modern veterinary practice or hospital nowadays. This includes also e-portals for online registration of new customers, online appointment bookings and e-payment portals. These are features that normally only professional companies can develop. Moreover, such electronic payment portals are excellent even for the often conservative veterinary practices, but they do require special licenses of the telecommunication providers as well as the bank. In veterinary practices that are located in border and frontier areas, the website might have to be bilingual to attract a higher customer volume. Website translation is often provided by professional website companies or can be arranged upon request. The extra costs usually pay off very well and provide additionally an excellent image of the veterinary practice. This can be especially helpful in border areas where pet owners may speak another language than English. This poses a new market segment for the veterinary practice, too.

Marketing and corporate identity is another important issue for modern veterinary practices and hospitals. Professional logos, stationary and marketing materials like flyers should be in the same design and display the corporate identity of the veterinary practice in a consistent form to the customers. This should be better contracted out-house as professional design reflects the professional image of the veterinary practice and hospital.

On the other hand, outsourcing recruitment is an entirely different issue. Several recruitment companies have specialized in veterinary human resources management and recruitment. First of all, every practice owner or practice manager should be very clear of what kind of new personnel he is looking for. A lot of possibilities exist for advertisement in specialized veterinary journals or websites. The practice own website can also be used as the platform for job advertisements, especially when talking about a large prestigious veterinary practice or specialist hospital. Specialized recruitment companies offer their services for sometimes up to twenty or twenty-five percent of the newly recruited staff first annual salary [6]. This is a huge sum, especially for a smaller practice, and it is questionable whether such an investment will really pay off. If the practice owner or manager is willing to use actively all possible tools for recruitment, then the high recruitment fees of specialized companies can be saved.

Before engaging in any outsourcing contract, it is advisable to get more information about the company. This includes information about [6]:

- Experience in veterinary issues
- References
- Finished work or projects
- Time in business
- Timeliness
- Pricing
- Fee structure or rates
- Contractual obligations

13.5. Conclusion

Ordering and supply-chain management has changed tremendously with the creation of the internet and e-business. Setting up of customer-friendly improvements like the hub- based chains, large wholesale veterinary suppliers have sped up processes that lead to 24 hours order and delivery cycles. Much to the advantage of the customers and thus also veterinary practices, this online ordering of medicines is very useful in the case of absolutely special and rarely used medicines that are prescribed to a selected pet with this condition. Moreover, medicines with short expiry dates can be stocked to a minimum and therefore, do not have to be discarded unused after they expire. This leads to many reduced inventories with the advantage of less bound invested money and fewer space requirements. However, the items in stock have to be properly stored and labeled to avoid damage or misuse. The inventory of pharmacy items and equipments like fixed asserts is taken on an annual basis.

Being heavily debated topic, outsourcing can be beneficial in few areas in the veterinary practice. These areas include especially accounting by a certified public accountant or marketing and printing. A good way of outsourcing is the use of specialized website design companies as nowadays many clients visit website to get updated information about the veterinary practice. Therefore, online appointment bookings and e-payment portals can prove extremely beneficial for practices to attract new clients and to open up markets among younger pet owners who are busily working.

References

[1]   Abu Aabed, A. (2007). Supply chain management. Outsourcing. *Assignment MBA Elective,* University of Strathclyde, Glasgow, UK.

[2]   Craig, D. and Willmott, P. (2005). *Outsourcing grows up.* McKinsey on Finance. Winter.

[3]   Embleton, P.R. and Wright, P.C. (1998). A guide to successful outsourcing. *Empowerment in Organizations.* Vol. 6, No. 3, pp. 94-106. http://www.emerald insight.com/Insight/ViewContentItem?ContentType=Article&hdAction=lnkhtml&cont entID=882437 . (Accessed on 30. December 2006).

[4]   Franceschini, F., Galetto, M., Pignatelli, A. and Varetto, M. (2003). Outsourcing: guidelines for a structured approach. Benchmarking: An International Journal. Vol. 10, No. 3, pp. 246-260. http://www.emeraldinsight.com/ Insight/ViewContentItem? ContentType=Article&hdAction=lnkhtml&contentID=843080. (Accessed on 30. December 2006).

[5]   Fink, D. (1994). A security framework for information systems outsourcing. Information Management & Computer Security. Vol.2, No. 4, pp. 3-8.http://www.emeraldinsight.com/Insight/ViewContentItem?ContentType=Article&hd Action=lnkhtml&contentID=862597 . (Accessed on 30. December 2006).

[6]   Goodman Lee, J. (2011).In practice. When not to do it yourself: Outsourcing in veterinary practice. *Compendium,* Vol. 33; No.1.

[7]   Gottschalk, P. and Solli-Sæther, H. (2006). Maturity model for IT outsourcing relationships. *Industrial Management & Data Systems.* Vol. 106, No. 2, pp. 200-

212.http://www.emeraldinsight.com/Insight/ViewContentItem?ContentType=Article&h dAction=Inkhtml&contentID=154880 . (Accessed on 30. December 2006).

[8]   Groucutt, J. and Griseri, P. (2004). *Mastering e-business.* Palgrave Master Series. New York.

[9]   Hurley, M. and Schaumann, F. (1997). KMPG survey: the IT outsourcing decision. Information Management & Computer Security. Vol. 5, No. 4, pp. 126-132. http://www.emeraldinsight.com/Insight/ViewContentItem?ContentType=Article&hdAc tion=Inkhtml&contentID=862695 . (Accessed on 30. December 2006).

[10]   Lacity, M. and Hirschheim, R. (1993). The information systems outsourcing bandwagon. Sloan Management Review. Vol. 35, No. 1, pp. 73-86.httpl//:www.research.ibm.com/journal/sj/431/rossref.html (Accessed on 30. December 2006).

[11]   Lankford, W.M. and Parsa, F. (1999). Outsourcing: a primer. Management Decision. Vol. 37, No. 4, pp. 310-316. http://www.emeraldinsight.com/Insight/View ContentItem?ContentType=Article&hdAction=Inkhtml&contentID=865066   . (Accessed on 30. December 2006).

[12]   Leavy, B. (2006). Supply chain effectiveness: strategy and integration. *Handbook of Business Strategy.* pp. 331-336.

[13]   Lee, M.K.O. (1996). IT outsourcing contracts: practical issues for 20. http://www. emeraldinsight.com/Insight/ViewContentItem?ContentType=Article&hdAction=Inkht ml&contentID=849812 . (Accessed on 30 December 2006).

[14]   Muller, M.G. (2007). Supply chain management elective. E-business and its influence on supply chain management— The rise of Dell. *Assignment MBA.* University of Strathclyde, Glasgow, UK.

[15]   Pfannenstein, L. and Tsai, R. (2004). Offshore outsourcing: current and future effects on American industry. *Information Systems Management.* Vol.21, No.4, pp. 72-80. http:// rit.edu/cje1611/OffshrOutsrcRvw.rtf (Accessed on 30. December 2006).

[16]   Rao, S.S. (2002). Making enterprises internet ready: e-business for process industries. *Work Study.* Vol. 51. No. 5. pp. 248-253.

[17]   Reynolds, J. (2004). The complete e-commerce book. 2nd ed. CMP Books. San Francisco. New York.

[18]   Shilcock, M. and Stutchfield, G.(2008). Veterinary practice management. *A practical guide.* 2nd ed. Saunders, Elsevier Ltd. Philadelphia.

[19]   Turban, E. and King, D. (2003). Introduction to e-commerce. *Person Education.* Prentice Hall. New Jersey.

Chapter 14

INFORMATION TECHNOLOGY MANAGEMENT AND INTERNET

ABSTRACT

Information technology has significantly advanced during the past decade. It is unthinkable to conduct any professional services and administrative work without the use of information technology nowadays. Moreover, the use of e-services and social networking sites has greatly enhanced the outreach to the general public and thus potential customers. Special computer programs for veterinary practices have become routine tools for veterinary practice management. However, still too many veterinary practices do not use information technology and internet to the maximum extent and thus lose out on a chance to increase their business.

The same applies to the use of websites as marketing tools. Therefore information technology and internet should be integrated to a much greater extent in the daily veterinary practice life.

14.1. INTRODUCTION

Since the 1990s, computers have found their way into our homes even in the developing countries and changed the life of people dramatically. Through the recent introduction of the internet, this new medium has led to fundamental personal and professional changes [4]. Companies had to face massive challenges in order to change their business way to answer to these modern e-commerce opportunities.

New e-business platforms have transformed traditional operations like supply chain management. However, some traditional ways stayed the same especially in logistics and order fulfillment procedures [13].

14.2. INFORMATION TECHNOLOGY

What is information technology? Despite the frequent use of this term, it is sometimes not fully understood what it really entails. The term" Information technology" or its abbreviation "IT" was first used in an article in Harvard Business review in 1958 [6]. It can be defined as "acquisition, processing, storage and dissemination of vocal, pictorial, textual and numerical information by a microelectronics-based combination of computing and telecommunications" [7].

Information technology includes all areas of information and technology management like computer software, computer hardware, information systems, processes as well as programming languages and data pools that have been visualized [14]. In recent years, the internet has emerged as an important business tool.

Despite the benefits of modern communication tools like internet, email and websites, those technologies have not yet found their way as routine administrative support in veterinary practices. A survey of the Royal College of Veterinary Surgeons in UK in 2006 revealed that only 15% or respondents use internet mainly at work and 35 % for work and at home. Although 82 % of respondents use email regularly, out of them only 57% have an email address at work [11].

14.3. VETERINARY SOFTWARE

In the early 1980s, veterinary software programs found their way into daily veterinary practice life. Nowadays more than 50% of veterinary practices use the help of computers [1] which is still alarmingly low compared to other modern businesses. Evidence-based medicine (EMR) has also been introduced in veterinary medicines.

Used in human medicine as a medical IT system, evidence-based medicine provides access to medical empirical information regarding treatments of various diseases [1]. In veterinary medicine, it is still used to a very minor extent as less than 1% of veterinary practitioners use such systems [1].

Although veterinary practices start to introduce specialized veterinary software in their work routine, they are frequently not using all its benefits. Research shows that less than 20% of software capabilities are actually used by veterinary practitioners [1]. This is even more unsatisfying when taking into consideration that one computer system can perform the work of two full-time staff in a medium-size veterinary practice [1].

14.3.1. Veterinary Software Content

How can the most suitable veterinary software be chosen for the veterinary practices? The best solution is a step-by-step approach that covers the topic software from all angles.

Following the answers to those questions, the practice owner or manager can decide which veterinary software program might be the most suitable. It can be either a small application for a small veterinary practice or a real business enterprise system for a large veterinary hospital or referral hospital. In case of a smaller veterinary practice with good growth potential, a modular veterinary software program can be helpful as it can grow together with the practice. Therefore the basic version can be bought in the beginning and further modules can be purchased following future expansion.

Table 14.1. Important questions for the right decision making about the veterinary practice software

Topics for decision-making	Important questions to decide about
Veterinary practice	• Size (small, medium, large)? • Use of software only for patient information data and billing? • Service enhancement through software? • Time saving through software?
Veterinary software	• Cost of software? • Demo version of software available? • Easy to use and navigate? • Modular system? • Future upgrades possible? • Content of software? • Desktop version or web-based application? • Server and hardware requirements for software?
Veterinary practice management	• Use of software for hospital management including accounting, inventory, HR and budget management? • Number of users? • Computer knowledge of staff? • Types of reports required? • Analysis of statistical business & medical data required? • Frequency of analysis?
Website	• Integration of software with website through use of e-services? • Online appointment bookings for veterinary services or consultation? • Online patient history for registered and approved clients
Vendor	• Visit for demonstration of software free of charge? • Modular software available? • Warranty duration? • Support services e.g. 24x7? • Training for the software and updates? • Cost of support services or support service contract? • Sale of software only or also hardware? • Maintenance contract? • Future upgrade free of charge or cost amount per man hour? • Possible internet hotline and problem fixing through external access?
Software users	• Computer literate? • Have used veterinary software before? • Understand that it is mandatory to use software?
External customers	• Does customer clientele use website for online appointment booking? • Mainly elderly people as customers? • Use of veterinary practice information emails helpful?

14.3.2. Database Management System

Data management can contain several topics depending upon the size and scope of practice. It may comprise normal data like patients' records, medical history and billing. However, good application software programs have inbuilt inventory management system and can be customized in a way that various other information like supplier details can be stored. Re-order stock levels can be established that provide a notification to the responsible employee about items to be reordered. Customization may also include the option to manage multiple batches and to use early expiry item first.

14.4. WEBSITE

A new market place has been established in the worldwide web. This leads to increased business opportunities and larger contact outreach to potential customer groups. It provides an ideal platform for veterinary practices to showcase their unique selling propositions and competitive advantages through specialized services to a large audience. This is especially helpful in bigger cities or highly populated areas. However, unfortunately veterinary practitioners do not use the website to the maximum extent as marketing tool. A well designed website does not only generate more customers but it enhances the convenience of pet owners to book appointments online, request some medications online or simply send a request at any time of day and night.

14.4.1. Preparation for Veterinary Website

The veterinary practice website can also inform about special campaign weeks or months that are dedicated e.g. for dental examination, flea and parasite treatment and geriatric examinations. News of the veterinary practice can be spread on the website news section and thus keep the pet owners engaged and in touch with the veterinary practice.

The size and content of the veterinary practice website depends on the size of the practice, its customer clientele and intended use of the website. It is highly useful to ask several questions before designing a website to ensure that the right website will be created.

After answering those questions, several next steps have to be decided. One of the most important ones is the choice of the website development vendor. Moreover, the web address or so-called Unique Resource Locator or URL has to be chosen and booked through one of the various web address providers. It is useful to choose a distinctive name or the name of the practice if available.

14.4.2. Veterinary Practice Website Content

The content of a good veterinary practice website has to include basic standard areas such as:

- *Home:* information about the veterinary practice in general
- *Services:* overview of the offered services with special emphasis on services that are exclusively provided by the practice and differentiate it from other competitors
- *News:* it is helping to enhance relationships with pet owners if latest news is published on the website. This may be a new continued professional education course that was successfully performed, introduction of new staff members or

acquisition of new equipments. It can also contain information about special marketing campaigns and special service offers.

Table 14.2. Important questions for the right decision making about the veterinary practice website

Topics for decision-making	Important questions to decide about
Veterinary practice	• Size (small, medium, large)? • Use of website as marketing tool or only general information about practice? • Service enhancement through website? • Increased business volume through website? • Outreach to new potential customer base through website? • Where the website be hosted?
Website	• Design by practice itself or specialized company? • Static or dynamic or interactive website? • Use of e-services? • Use of e-payment portal? • Integration of software with website? • Online appointment bookings to be merged with veterinary software appointment schedules? • Interactive system e.g. for requesting medicines etc? • Cost of website? • Demo or dummy version of similar website available? • Easy to use and navigate? • Modular system? • Can be upgraded in future? • Content of website? • Content management and updates to be done by vendor or practice? • Server and hardware requirements for website?
Veterinary practice management	• Use of integrated website and software solution for hospital management? • Number of internal users? • Computer knowledge qualification of staff? • Analysis of statistical business data required? • Frequency of analysis? • IT knowledge in-house for website updates?
Vendor	• Visit for demonstration of already designed websites free of charge? • Modular website available? • Warranty duration? • Support services e.g. 24x7? • Cost of support services or support service contract? • Maintenance contract? • Future upgrade free of charge or cost amount? • Possible internet hotline and problem fixing through external access?
External customers	• Large number of potential new customers in catchment area? • Does customer clientele use website for online appointment booking? • Mainly elderly and less computer literate people as customers? • Mainly busy working people as customers? • Use of veterinary practice information via website and emails helpful? • Requests of seeing pet patient records online?

- *Forms:* Various forms as per requirements of the practice either for integration with software application, enquiry and/or feedback
- *Location:* apart from the general location description, it is good to provide a location map eventually with GPS data information
- *Contact information:* this should include name, address, phone and fax numbers, email address and emergency number

Optional are the following information:

- *Staff information:* customers might not be able to see all staff members. This section can provide them with information about staff members, their individual areas of expertise, employee of the month selection (if available). Thus animal owners get more integrated in the veterinary practice team as it becomes visible for them.
- *General information:* about correct pet husbandry, diseases and disease prevention as well as information on vaccinations, regular examinations and spaying and neutering procedures.
- *Online patient records:* although this part of a website will be reserved mainly for larger veterinary practices and hospitals, it can reduce the number of phone calls of concerned pet owners asking for the health condition of their pet, e.g. after surgery or in boarding kennels. Through the availability of electronic online patient records, the owners can receive the information he needs in a convenient and time efficient way.
- *Lost and found page:* veterinary practices are often informed when a pet has gone missing. Therefore it is an excellent customer service to have a lost and found page on the website where owner information of missing pets can be made public and thus enhances the chances to reallocate a found pet.
- *Photo gallery:* this can include photos of the practice facilities as pet owners are normally not allowed to enter the main practice facilities like surgeries. It can also contain pictures of successful surgeries, beautiful before and after grooming photos, pictures of adopted pets and happy endings etc.
- *E-services:* please refer to below part in this chapter
- *E-payments:* please refer to below part in this chapter

14.4.3. Website Hosting Sites

Another decision that needs to be taken is the location where the website will be hosted. There are different possibilities for site hosting. One host site is the practice itself if required hardware servers and resources are available. This will, however, mainly apply to larger veterinary practices. It is also possible to host predesigned website from personal computers which is suitable for smaller practices, too.

In many cases, the use of Internet Service Provider's (ISP) host site is preferred as they can be rented out for a lower rate comparatively. Although the space on the respective servers is rented out, the content of the website can be managed by the practice with being fully in control using website's content management software [5].

Some specialized website design companies provide the possibility to host website on their servers but in most cases they retain the control over the web content. It then requires the company to make changes and update the website content as this cannot be done by the veterinary practice itself. However, the website can be managed using online content management of the website if available.

14.5. E-BUSINESS (ELECTRONIC BUSINESS)

In its simplest form, the conduct of business on the Internet is called e-Business (electronic business). Being a more generic term than eCommerce, e-Business includes also servicing customers and collaborating with business partners apart from just buying and selling [2]. IBM was one of the first to use the term in 1997 [5].

14.5.1. General Information About E-Business

In our modern times, e-business has become a household term. Almost everybody is talking now about e-business but it is not always clear what it really means. However, many times the term e-business and e-commerce are used in an identical way. E-commerce is defined as the value exchange through internet between companies and their respective employees, customers and partners without time or geographic borders [4]. The term e-business is including e-commerce, but has a wider application by taking the macro-environmental. Those outside PESTEL factors include political, economical, social, technological, environmental and legal influences. In the supply chain management world, the e-procurement is the on-line purchase of raw material and supply. Moreover, the terms internet and World Wide Web are not synonyms as the internet means the general computer network used for data transfer. The World Wide Web is defined as the specific browser based services with URLs and HTML for all kinds of text, image and audio files [4, 8].

Due to the convenience, availability, and world-wide reach of the internet, many companies, organizations and practices have already discovered how to use the internet successfully [5]. Their numbers are increasing constantly which applies at a much slower pace for veterinary practices, too.

The value of e-business transactions have tremendously increased in past years. Whereas the volume of e-business in 1999 covered US$ 150.15bn, it jumped in 2005 to staggering US$ 530.0bn. This indicates not only commercial value, but also stresses the importance of e-business in our modern world [4]. The Asia/Pacific region is one of the fastest growing regions especially in global B2B trade [11].

As global interface the internet provides the chance of e-business between different groups and individuals. Business can be done from Customer-to-Business (C2B) and Business-to-Customer (B2C). Moreover, it can be performed on the same level like Customer-to-Customer (C2C) or Business-to-Business (B2B). A growing potential with forecasted rise in the future is the Government-to-Citizen (G2C) business area [4, 8].

In the process industries, e-business is gaining wider importance through streamlined business processes, web based services for internal business process support and interactive portals e.g. with suppliers. Moreover, supply chains will become integrated to provide reliable information for suppliers and business partners as well as real time systems will come in place. The future of process industry e-business is becoming more customer-oriented with online exchanges and enhanced customer services like order placing or tracking through the internet website. This interconnectivity between suppliers, manufacturers, distributors and customers has increased the dynamics of process industries. It has changed the way some processes are performed, too [11]. Nowadays, the security built into today's browsers and with digital certificates is now available for individuals and companies from certificate issuer like Verisign [5, 9]. Therefore, much of the previous strong concerns about the security of business transaction on the Web have subsided and e-business is speeding up tremendously [5, 9].

14.5.2. E-Services and E-Payment Portals

Modern life leads to customers with busy time schedules, which have less and less time and therefore require more convenience services. Veterinary practices can help in this by through an excellent interactive website that allows e-services and e-payments.

E-services are very useful and powerful customer satisfaction tools. Especially e-services used for online appointment bookings are very customer friendly as this saves considerable time for busy animal owners and receptionists alike.

E-payment services provide the possibility to pay for services or products via credit card or external payment portals. This requires a secure internet line that has to adhere to the latest internet security standards. Moreover, the veterinary practice requires an online payment bank account where all online payments will be transferred to. It should not be forgotten that the banks will take a certain percentage of the payment as their own charge which leads to a slight reduction in the final payment for the veterinary practice. However, online payment is a fast and reliable tool that helps the veterinary practitioner to get his money without delays. E-payment services are especially helpful for pet owners who use pet boarding facilities in veterinary practices with pet pick-up and drop-off services. E-payment portals can also be used by busy working pet owners who send their pet through pick-up service for an examination to the veterinary practice. Moreover, they make it easier for pet owners to pay for e.g. medicine against parasites or vitamins that can be then send to them by mail or delivered to their doorstep. If the veterinary practice has a pet shop, the online payment service can also be used for the sale of merchandising items.

14.5.3. E-Marketing

Electronic marketing or the so-called eMarketing is the application of marketing principles and techniques via electronic media and more specifically the Internet. Frequently interchanged, the terms eMarketing, Internet marketing and online marketing, can often be used as synonyms terms [10]. Its ultimate aim is to enhance the reputation of the brand, to get new customers and to keep old customers loyal. A major advantage for the veterinary practice is the fact that e-marketing can be considered as not expensive marketing tool. The return on investment (ROI) from eMarketing can far exceed that of traditional marketing strategies when it has been implemented correctly [10].Moreover, it can reach wide audiences and open potential markets.

14.6. SOCIAL NETWORKING SITES

Social networking site like Facebook, twitter or LinkedIn are becoming part of modern lifestyles of hundreds of millions of people. This can be profitable for veterinary practitioners as those social networking sites can be used as marketing tools for veterinary practices, too. Putting the veterinary practice on those networking sites and feeding them with news and information can be helpful in gaining exposure to a wider customer clientele, especially the younger one, and to spread the reputation of the practice.

Social networking sites can also be used in the human resources parts of the veterinary practices to filter job applicants. It can be extremely useful to check upon potential job candidates on those networking sites as this can provide very good information about them. For example, there is no need to employ a new staff member who puts negative comments about his previous employer on his social networking site. But those sites can also provide useful information about positive aspects of job seekers who worked in animal welfare projects etc.

14.7. EMAIL

The use of electronic mails or emails in the veterinary practice is manifold. It is one of the modern communication and messaging tools. Despite its ease of use, email etiquette should be followed. This includes the subject topic as headline, short but professional messages and no personal comments in a business email. It is very professional if all employees in the veterinary practice follow the same email signature as corporate identity.

Emails can also be very helpful in customer relations services as pet owners can send emails with enquiries or booking to veterinary practices. They can be used as email reminders to customers for e.g. vaccination reminders. Moreover, emails serve as information tool for new services, promotional campaigns and newsletters.

Important emails should be stored in a safe place as they might be required later. Large attachments are better saved in a special document folder in order to keep the email inbox size in its limits.

14.8. INFORMATION AND INTERNET SECURITY

14.8.1. Information Security Risks

Accidental security problems can be caused by human errors and form the largest cause for damage to information security. This can be either through inaccurate data entry in the database or failure to make correct backup. Moreover, information security issues can arise when the employee is overloaded with his task and incapable to fulfill it correctly [2].

Unauthorized access and use of confidential data poses another risk to information security. This is less applicable to possible hackers as their numbers are very small compared to possible threats inside the business entity, namely through employees [2].

Another problem can happen through sabotage of an individual. Although not very common, this should be taken into consideration in cases of termination of staff as they might seek revenge and leave the biggest possible damage. Therefore it might be advisable to remove terminated staff from any access to information systems and data base with immediate effect in order to protect the system [2] and subsequent valuable practice data.

Information security can be breached through theft which can be divided in physical theft and data theft. This might be applicable again in the case of terminated employees who might like to take the customer address data base with them and then set up their own veterinary practice in the same area as their previous employer [2].

14.8.2. Information Systems Security Controls

Breaches in the information systems security can be avoided by recovery mechanisms that can retrieve backup data. For larger veterinary hospitals, a backup site or disaster recovery (DR) site might be useful on which the copy of the complete data material is housed. This may include data processing facilities, hardware, software as well as up-to-date data files. In case of emergency, the processing can be switched to the DR site without loss of valuable time to ensure a smooth continuation of the work process without interruption. The recovery of business data is essential and requires well planned procedures through the so-called business contingency planning. Full or partial Backups should be taken routinely e.g. daily, weekly or monthly depending on the amount of data to be stored. Backup tapes with huge storage are commonly used backup media these days. Useful are external hard drives as they have a huge storage volume, too and are relatively low priced. One copy of backup data should always be stored outside the veterinary practice in a safe location that not all backup data copies will be destroyed in case of fire, floods or other unexpected damage. One possibility of storing backup data in a safe way is the use of three different backup storage facilities where data are stored on a rotating set up of backup disks or hard drives. This creates three different versions of the same data stored at any time. However, it should not be forgotten that only approximately 5% of computer users know how to make a correct backup. Therefore responsible employees in the veterinary practice should be trained in correct backup procedures [2].

Regular audits of data, hardware and software are other helpful tool to prevent damage to information systems. This leads to a good overview of available data and information system parts and may reduce unauthorized use of systems by employees, e.g. through illegal software installations [2].

Use of passwords with various authorization levels for computer-based information systems can help to restrict unauthorized access and provide only those areas with access that the employees needs to work with. Although commonly used, it is well-known that passwords easily get exchanged among employees. Therefore passwords should not be used as ultimate security tool on which to rely on solely [2].

Another important and very effective tool for information systems security is the introduction of formal and comprehensive policies on security. They can be set up following international standards and contain usually the areas of acceptable and unacceptable use of information systems. Moreover, they include also sanctions for the case that employees do not comply with the security policies. Well publicized and enforced, formal security policies can be regarded as simple and effective and can be used in every veterinary practice [2].

14.8.3. Internet Security Risks

The main internet security risk is caused by computer viruses that create huge financial and data losses to modern businesses worldwide. A variety of different viruses exist and new ones are created on daily basis. However, the virus can only be transmitted through email attachments that, once opened, infect the computer. Other possibilities of virus transmission are personal memory sticks or disks of employees that they bring from their personal computers at home to office and which are infected with illegal software or downloads from the internet. Some employees also use the internet in the office for their private use and might go to infected websites [2].

But internet security is not only affected by viruses. In recent years, the existence of worms and Trojans has risen tremendously with major financial business damages. Worms can be described as small programs that have the potential to change or overwrite data pieces while moving through the computer. In contrast, Trojans look like legitimate programs that try to get access to the computer systems. Trojans have the capability to incorporate the key logging facility which means they can record all entries on the keyboard including passwords and contents of outgoing e-mail messages [2].

A new type of internet threat is spyware that may affect both, office and home computer users. Often distributed as so-called adware which means advertising supported software, spywares can be provided by companies as advertisement to no or low charge. They can capture and record confidential data and monitors the user's activities without the knowledge or consent of the computer user and then transit the report to their producers [2].

14.9. CONCLUSION

Veterinary software programs are a tremendous help for all practice types. They speed up the workflow and aid in correct and precise practice management. Before purchasing special veterinary practice management software, the individual needs and requirements of the practice have to be identified and considered to invest in the right product as a wide range of veterinary software programs are available nowadays.

The introduction of internet, website and e-business has fundamentally transformed not only the general business world, but also the veterinary practice life. Their use leads to a variety of new business opportunities that can be of great benefit for the veterinary practice. One of them is the wide outreach to a new group of potential customers that are internet savvy and expect e-business to ease their life. Another advantage of websites is the use of electronic appointments bookings and e-payment portals. Websites have a positive impact on marketing the veterinary practice's services and facilities as well as to provide additional information about animal diseases and their prevention.

Despite previous concerns with internet security, especially while performing financial transaction, modern security enhancements through digital certificates are available nowadays. They improve internet security to a high level. However, still some residual risks exist mainly though internet viruses, worms or Trojan software that can never be ruled out fully.

REFERENCES

[1] Ackermann, Lowell (2007). Blackwell's five-minute veterinary practice management consult. *Blackwell Publishing*. Iowa. USA.

[2] Alexandrou, M. (2011). eBusiness definition. Internet directory. Infolific. http://infolific.com/technology/definitions/internet-dictionary/ebusiness (Accessed on August 23rd, 2011).

[3] Bocij, P., Chaffey, D., Greasley, A. and Hickie, S. (2006). Business information systems.Technology, development & management for the e-business.3rd. ed. Prentice Hall.Financial Times.

[4] Groucutt, J. and P.Griseri (2004). *Mastering e-business. Palgrave Master Series*. New York.

[5] Kumar, K. (2011). Personal communication.

[6] Leavitt, H.J. and Whisler, P.E. (1958). Management in the 1990s. *Harvard Business Review*. pp. 41-48.

[7] Longley, D. and Shain, M. (1985). Dictionary of information technology.2nd ed. Macmillan Press.

[8] Muller, M.G. (2007). Supply chain management elective. E-business and its influence on supply chain management— The rise of Dell. Assignment MBA Elective. University of Strathclyde, Glasgow, UK.

[9] Nelson, T.D. (2000). E-business. (electronic business). http://searchcio.techtarget.com/definition/e-business. (Accessed on August 20th, 2011).

[10] Quirk (2006). What is eMarketing and how is it better than traditional marketing? Chapter 1. November. pp. 1-6. http://www.quirk.biz/cms/801.emarketingone-chapone.pdf (Accessed on August 20th, 2011).

[11] Rao, S.S. (2002). Making enterprises internet ready: e-business for process industries. *Work Study*. Vol. 51.No. 5. pp. 248-253.

[12] RCVS (2006). The UK veterinary profession in 2006. The findings of a survey of the professionconducted by the Royal College of Veterinary Surgeons.

[13] Reynolds, J. (2004). The complete e-commerce book. 2nd ed. CMP Books. San Francisco. New York.

[14] Wikipedia (2011). Information technology. http://en.wikipedia.org/wiki/information_technology#CITEREFLLongleyShain1985 (Accessed on February 5th 2011).

Chapter 15

MARKETING

ABSTRACT

Marketing in the veterinary practice helps to get information about the practice and its services out to the clients and interested potential new clients. Increased competition forces practices to become more pro-active in their marketing approach to reach out to a wider range of interested animal owners. Good marketing requires well-designed marketing campaigns that can create major benefit for the veterinary practice which is explained in detail in this chapter. A part of marketing is the setting up of corporate identity and branding to give the practice a special look and logo. The unique selling proposition of the practice has to be identified and visualized to the potential customers. The marketing campaign exists of external and internal strategies with inclusion of an excellent website. Mistakes in marketing have to be avoided in order to protect and to create a positive image of the veterinary practice.

15.1. INTRODUCTION

Marketing has been defined as "The management process … responsible for identifying, anticipating and satisfying customer requirements profitably" [4, p.119].

Despite a lot of prejudices against modern marketing [5], it is a valuable help in the veterinary's strategy regarding customer requirement's information, profit [10] as well as customer's education about important veterinary services [7]. Moreover, marketing should be performed in the form of marketing concepts, which are "the achievements of corporate goals through meeting and exceeding customer needs better than the competition" [5, p.911]. However, marketing should not be mistaken with advertising, which is defined as "any paid form of non-personal communication of ideas or products in the prime media, i.e. television, the press, posters, cinema and radio, the internet and direct marketing" [5, p.905].

15.2. GENERAL VETERINARY PRACTICE MARKETING

Marketing covers a wide range of activities, including market research, marketing planning, market positioning, sales, public relations, advertising, consumer behavior research, pricing and managing products and services [5,10]. Due to the increased competition in the veterinary practice sector, practices need to become much more pro-active and reach out to potential customers and their specific requirements. This can be achieved by well-planned and co-ordinate marketing strategies [10] considering the four P's of marketing, namely price, place, product and promotions. However, in some European countries like Germany and Austria, advertising of the personal veterinary practice or its services is not allowed by law for veterinarians [8].

New veterinary practices require a pro-active and comprehensive marketing strategy for both, services and products, in the opening phase like advertisement, newspaper articles featuring the practice and it special services as well as flyers. Flyers can be distributed close to all major shops, supermarkets, schools and large residential areas. The website of the newly opened practice has to provide interactive e-marketing and must be well linked for easy-access [6].

15.2.1. Benefits of Marketing Strategies for Veterinary Practices

The benefits of marketing for veterinary practices are manifold. On one hand, marketing helps to cause a change to the other competing practices by positively and pro-actively approaching potential customers. It leads to a higher profile of the practice and the veterinary profession in general. Professional marketing offers a platform to advertise about new services or specializations of the practices which are not known to the pet owners yet [10]. This might attract even new customers if the marketing tools that are used meet their needs and requirements. On the other hand, it might keep the customer clientele loyal and interested in the practice. These marketing outcomes may lead to increased income through services and products. The profitability of a practice can also be raised by launching a marketing campaign during the slower months of the year thus targeting pet owners directly who would not go to the veterinarian during this time [7]. One example for such campaign is the "Month of the Mouth" for dental examination and cleaning or the "Week of Nutrition" for correct feeding advice and nutritional information of pets. There is no restriction for fantasy in creating special marketing promotion campaigns. Many veterinary practices do not use such campaigns to the full extent as they underestimate the financial impact of such campaigns. Moreover, marketing strengthens the customer bond to the practice and thus enhances the reputation and caretaker image of the veterinary practice.

15.2.2. Budgeting for Marketing

The budget for marketing is the tool for controlling and monitoring the expenses. The amount of this budget is connected with the resources available and the set goals and objectives. Moreover, marketing budgets are usually a percentage of the projected sales of this year [2]. However, for a veterinary practice, it is required to find out the correlation between certain marketing tools like newsletter or reminder cards and increased service income. The same applies to the products sold. Marketing tools, which are very well accepted by the clientele can be extended and improved.

15.3. CORPORATE IDENTITY AND BRANDING

Corporate identity and branding are commonly used terms in the modern business world. Branding describes the process of distinguishing products from competitors. This can be either through a special logo, name or design [5]. In contrast, corporate identity comprises the aims and values of an organization that is represented to the outside world through the visual cohesive images [5]. This includes also behavior, communication and dress codes.

A highly important part of the well-planned marketing strategy is the clear visibility of the corporate identity of the practice because "image is vital for your success" [7, p.36]. This can be achieved by the corporate design which includes the practice logo, business cards and stationary. Special practice flyers and practice brochures will also help to reach out to a wider audience [7]. However, corporate identity is not only the corporate design, but also the corporate communication and behavior [8]. Corporate communication includes the clear and consistent communication strategy of practice staff towards the customer to show the professionalism of the practice. All messages given to the customers must be unified as otherwise they will not trust that the practice will provide excellent services for them. Moreover, the corporate behavior of the practice staff is another very important feature of the practice corporate identity [8]. This includes the same attitude and behavior towards the pet owners as to the pets themselves. An excellent corporate behavior can result in a positive image and thus competitive advantage to other veterinary practices.

A good and distinctive logo is very crucial for the corporate identity and marketing success. It may be representing the animal species that the veterinary practice is specialized in, but it can be also funny and funky. Humorous pet motives are especially attractive for small animal owners.

15.4. MARKETING STRATEGIES

15.4.1. Unique Selling Proposition/ Point (USP)

The concept of the unique selling proposition or point (USP) was first introduced as marketing in advertising campaigns in the early 1940s. It means that the USP is a proposition that is unique, and it aims to convince potential customers to change brands. In advertising the USP means that the customers get the information about specific benefits when buying the proposed product. It also indicates that no other competitor can offer the same product or services. Moreover, the USP must have a strong meaning in order to influence customers on larger scales [9].

15.4.2. External Marketing Strategies

A very valuable and attractive external marketing tool is the practice newsletter which is often published on a quarterly basis. This newsletter has to be designed and printed in a professional way as this directly reflects the image of the practice. Their main aim is to provide an information platform for the practice's clients and to inform about new services and products the practice has to offer [6]. New staff members can be introduced to the clientele [10]. This makes customers feel comfortable as they will feel they are integrated in the practice thus strengthening the client – veterinary practice bonds. Moreover, the newsletter helps the practice to market new machines and equipment or inform about seasonal requirements for pets like deworming [7, 8].

Advertising aims to provide information about the existence of the veterinary practice, its services and location. It can be done in the yellow pages phone directory or the directory of the veterinary associations [10]. The most important area for advertising is the catchment area of the practice but also the radius around that.

Most pet owners do not only love their pet, but also like and enjoy fashionable pet accessories. A very special way of promoting the practice is the special design of pet bandannas with logo, name and phone number thus making not only the pet and its owner proud, but also providing good advertising for the practice [7].

Cards reminding of due vaccinations or re-checks are another tool of external marketing. Although not all clients will respond to them, still they will remember the practice. For those pet owners who respond by bringing their pet for a visit, the card has paid off very well [7, 10]. Healthcare programs like dog puppy or kitten parties, dental check-ups or geriatric check-ups do not only generate more income, but they also reach out to increase awareness and bonding with the clients [10].

Another new medium for wide-reaching marketing is the internet website. Many practices have started to have their own web page with all information regarding address, location, opening hours, services provided, products offered, general information about diseases, staff directory, sections of lost and found pets, virtual tours and news. Moreover, e-shops or their links on practice websites are becoming increasingly popular [10]. This is explained in detail in chapter 14 "Information technology" in this book.

Despite being unknown five years ago, social media have an ever increasing influence on the private but also business world. One way of getting more visibility to potential customers and increasing customer loyalty and retention is using social media. It has been reported that companies engaged in social media saw an increase of 18% in one year. In contrast, companies that did not engage in social media posted an average revenue decline of 6% in the same period of time [3]. Veterinary practice being on social-networking sites might can create larger visibility and enhance identification with clients with the customers, especially of the younger generation.

15.4.3. Internal Marketing Strategies

A very valuable tool for internal marketing is the education of the customers by distributing information leaflets about some diseases or disease prevention during the waiting time or following a consultation. They feature again the practice logo, name and address [7]. Information leaflets can be self-designed to cater for a special customer clientele or can be ordered from the veterinary association or chambers.

Videos about disease prevention are usually provided by the pharmaceutical industry to promote their products. Shown in the reception and waiting area, they might be useful not only for an increased knowledge of the pet owner [7], but also to increase the sale of products like for flea prevention.

Another way of marketing the services and practices internally is the photo gallery or video of the practice facility. This helps to keep animal owners busy during their waiting time by watching specially made movies announcing about the practice and its service. Furthermore, a good marketing tool is the employees of the month photo with his or her name and designation. Moreover, pet owners love to have the most beautiful pet of the month contest with photo in the reception area, especially if it is their own pet. A certificate and small reward (e.g. pet accessory, special dog biscuits or voucher for a free consultation) should be given away for this pet, which will be highly attractive for pet owners.

15.5. MISTAKES IN MARKETING AND ADVERTISING

The main marketing mistake is to lose touch with the customer base. Customers are the most important part of the existing and future veterinary business. If they feel less valued or neglected, then they might decide to go to another veterinary practice. One very helpful tool to avoid this problem is the regular distribution of newsletters to the customers [1] as mentioned above.

One of the main advertising mistakes is the advertising of a low price without emphasizing the value of services. This will only attract customers who are looking for the cheapest price and do not appreciate good services and therefore, pose a wrong market segment for the veterinary practice. Such customers will never be loyal as they will always go to another practice if they get a cheaper price even. They do not care if the services might not be up to standards [1].

Another major advertising mistake is the advertising of a percentage for services. This will lead to a "x % reduction" for a service which is very difficult for customers to relate to as they are usually not aware of the prices of individual services. It is much easier for them to get clear figures [1] like "bring your pet for vaccination and get the examination for free" or "get US$ 20 off for the first dental cleaning of your pet". This will increase the customer clientele, and they will return as loyal customers when the veterinary service had been satisfying, and they enjoyed the positive atmosphere in the veterinary practice.

A further mistake is not to stress the competitive advantage and unique selling proposition of the veterinary practice in advertisements and especially in advertisement headlines [1]. Customers need to realize the difference between your practice and other veterinary practices. This can be done through professional specializations like dentistry, alternative medicine, surgery or feline internal medicine but also through excellent customer service, no waiting times or home visits. Special dedicated programs for pets can be advertised in those specialized areas to let customers understand their benefits in visiting a respective veterinary practice.

15.6. CONCLUSION

Marketing can be an extremely important strategic tool to increase the veterinary practice income and to strengthen the bonds between the customers and the veterinary practice. However, it must be executed in a professional way and according to the individual needs and requirements of the veterinary practice. It is imperative that the practice owner or practice manager first needs to understand the customer base to address the marketing campaign according to their interest. Marketing should not be regarded as an ad-hoc campaign when the income is down but rather planned well ahead on a yearly basis considering slower visit times during the year, holidays etc.. Corporate identity should be set up carefully in order not be changed repeatedly as this only leads to the confusion of customers. Streamlined behavior and dealing with customers in the same unified message by all practice staff helps to create an excellent marketing and enhances the reputation of the practice very effectively. In the same time, it is the most cost-effective marketing tool available.

REFERENCES

[1]   Danie, M.Y. (2008). Own a veterinary practice? 5 costly marketing mistakes you must not ignore. http://ezinearticles.com/Own-a-Veterinary-Practice?-5-Costly-Marketing-Mistakes-You-Must-Not-Ignore&id=1336613 (Accessed on February 4th, 2011).

[2]   Gillespie, A. (1998). *Advanced Business Studies through diagrams.* Oxford University Press. UK.

[3]   Goodman Lee, J. (2011).In practice. When not to do it yourself: Outsourcing in veterinary practice. *Compendium,* Vol. 33; No.1.

[4]   Hindle, T. and Thomas, M. (1994). The economist books: Pocket marketing. 2nd ed. Penguin Group. Hamondsworth, Middlesex, England.

[5]   Jobber, D. (2004). Principles and practice of marketing. 4th ed. McGraw-Hill Int. Ltd. Berkshire, UK.

[6]   Müller, M.G. and Abu Aabed, A. (2007). Guidelines for setting up a small and medium size enterprise. MBA Thesis, University of Strathclyde. Graduate School of Business. Glasgow, UK.

[7]   Oppermann, M. (1999). The art of veterinary practice management. *Veterinary Medicine Publishing Group.* Lenexa, Kansas, USA.

[8]   Ouwerkerk, M. and Schlegel, H. (1997). Erfolgreiche Praxisführung für den Tierarzt: Praxismanagament/ Praxismarketing. Hannover. Schlütersche GmbH.

[9]   Reeves, R. (1961). Reality in advertising. New York, Alfred. A. Knopf, LCCN 61007118. http://en.wikipedia.org/wiki/Unique_selling_proposition. (Accessed on February 4th, 2011).

[10]   Shilcock, M. and Stutchfield, G.(2008). Veterinary practice management. *A practical guide.* 2nd ed. Saunders, Elsevier Ltd. Philadelphia.

Chapter 16

LEADERSHIP AND EMPOWERMENT

ABSTRACT

Leadership and empowerment are very popular terms in modern business management. They are fixed parts in modern manager training programs, but have also started to find their way in veterinary executive education through special training programs. With regard to leadership, the old question arises whether leaders are born or made, which is a very disputed among researchers. Certain skills and competencies can be learnt in training programs, but character traits cannot be taught in leadership courses. Empowerment in the veterinary practice may lead to major improvements in productivity, team work and consequently, profits. However, this might only work when employees are ready to take increased responsibilities and leaders accept to share their power. This chapter sheds light on the use of leadership and empowerment in the daily veterinary practice routine.

16.1. INTRODUCTION

Where does leadership find its place in the veterinary practice management? In a fast changing, highly dynamic veterinary world, leadership is required to face the challenges of those changes. Different levels of leadership can be experienced in general business companies but can be used in veterinary practices, too. Veterinary employees in important higher ranking positions definitely require leadership qualities. This applies especially to practice owners, managers and head veterinarians. Leadership levels can be divided upon different competencies. But can leadership be really learnt or is a leader born as a leader? The question "Are leaders born or made?" can be traced back centuries ago to the old Greek philosophers and is under heavy debate until today [20]. When entering this question into the internet search machine Google, a stunning number of 10,200,000 results can be found. Researchers found that certain leadership traits and skills can be allocated to genes and thus being inherited [25]. In contrast, some people believe that leaders are only shaped through external influences, experiences and opportunities [23]. A combination of both has also been stated [20].

16.2. LEADERSHIP IN VETERINARY PRACTICES

Nowadays, a large variety of different leadership programs attracts hopeful managers with the aim to become leaders. They are designed in various ways in order to develop certain leadership skills. However, inherited characteristics of good leaders like intelligence, charisma and inspiration [3] can never be learnt. This leads to the conclusion that leaders are born, but certain leadership skills can be developed through training. However, through training alone and without any genetic determination, no leader will be made [29]. In the veterinary field, leadership programs have not yet found widespread acceptance as veterinarians do not see themselves as leaders. The general concepts of leadership are not yet fully integrated in the veterinary life and only start to emerge slowly.

16.2.1. Research on Leadership

What makes a good leader? Researchers which support the theory that leaders are born believe that the genes and childhood are the major contributing factors for development of leadership. Moreover, they state that "the "right" genes and the "right" family are relatively rare, and that this rarity explains why we see so few leaders" [15, p.19]. It is said that leaders are born, and managers are made because each group has certain distinct competencies [24]. Some attributes regarded as outwards signs of leadership are height, energy, a commanding voice as well as intelligence and assertiveness. Intelligence and physical energy are genetically determined. Moreover, a lot of personality traits like the so-called social potency which determines a masterful and forceful leader have been identified to be at least 61% of genetic origin. The same applies to harm avoidance and risk taking being other leadership criteria [15]. Other genetic studies have found out that most of the leadership dimensions are inherited as well as the two higher-level factors. Those resemble the form of transactional and transformational leadership. The former is additively inherited to 48% whereas the latter can be explained by non additive and therefore, dominant heritability to 59%. Even multivariate analysis result in large overlaps of the genes being responsible for the leadership dimensions [25].

Childhood experiences are also highly important in leadership, especially with regard to the development of language usage and skills as well as intelligence, understanding and dealing with other people. The childhood conditioning has direct influence on the child's ability of strategic thinking, articulation, motivation and alignment of others. This relates also to self-esteem and the capacity and need for social role taking, which can be supported by parents serving as catalysts [15]. The main development in the childhood can be found in the first seven years. Moreover, early signs of leadership might be indicated through taking responsibilities in leading positions at school, university or in sports teams [20].

In contrast, a majority of leadership researchers favors that leaders are made [23]. The origin of leadership can be learnt during the life through specific experiences or opportunities. Those experiences and opportunities can be work-related, or arise from hardship, education as well as certain role models and mentoring. It is widely believed that the relatively few numbers of leaders derive from neglected development rather than potential abilities. Moreover, formal training as well as experiences in certain projects and development jobs are also contributing to the shaping of leaders. However, motivation has a great impact on the development of leaders as through lack of motivation to take over hardships and responsibilities the number of leaders will be limited. Leaders must be unconventional, break out of routines and take risks being a feature of personal development [15]. The major impact on the making of leaders is the learning process first on the professional basis and then on the peoples' motivational and behavioral level [35].

There are also opinions that favor the combination of leaders who are born and made, too [20]. Although there exist several inherited personality or character traits, intelligence is regarded as the major contributing factors for potential future leaders [5]. Up to 80% of leadership qualities might be acquired through learning, even from previous failures or negative experiences. The overcoming of those failures and the ability to learn from them, even on a life-long basis, contributes effectively to leadership skills. Good leaders are open to new experiences and are looking for further development opportunities to acquire new skills [5]. The right environment is also helpful in developing leaders and leaderships [21].

16.2.2. Effectiveness of Leadership Training Programs

The question arises of leadership programs can be considered as useful in general and might they be applicable for aspiring veterinary leaders? A lot of debate about the usefulness and effectiveness of leadership programs is currently going on. It has been stated that leadership training is not a useful tool to transform people into leaders [12] because personal traits like integrity and credibility as well as trust cannot be learnt through training programs [26]. In contrast, it has been argued that leadership can be developed under certain conditions like the desire to learn, focusing on special leadership behavior and the practicing of the learnt skills [20].

Leadership programs are offered nowadays already for teenagers, e.g. by the Princeton Center for Leadership Training in order to achieve a positive peer influence [32]. Moreover, those programs are intended to break psychological barriers to effective leadership. Those barriers are low self-esteem and self-confidence as well as fear of failure and thinking 'inside the box' as well as negative stress. Through the techniques taught in leadership programs those barriers can be overcome [18,20]. Effective leadership programs include working relationships, 360 degree feedback as well as formal mentoring and action learning whereas conventional learning methods are not very much widespread [20]. Therefore, leadership programs like the one from The Leadership Trust combine leadership training with extreme outdoor experiences to achieve the application of leadership techniques under immoderate situations and physical pressure. This is intended to raise self-awareness and self-discipline, both fundamental key success factors for strong leadership. Some techniques are desensitization, reinforcement theory and psychological enactment. Moreover, acquisition of social skills and group dynamics may help to become leaders [18, 20]. Leadership programs do not only cater for high-level executives, but also for lower level managers. Criteria for entering some leadership training programs are not academic qualifications, but personal interest and professional experience. Even long-distance learning has found its way into leadership training programs [10].

The approach of the United Nations University and its International Leadership Academy seems to go in the right direction with the opinion that although leadership itself cannot be learnt the skills associated with leadership can be acquired [20] or improved through training [4]. This stands in line with some leadership training programs that acknowledge that certain elements of leadership can be taught [28].

In veterinary medicine, leadership programs slowly find their way into the university curricula, especially in the USA. Veterinary medicine colleges like Washington State University offer special AVMA Veterinary Leadership Experience programs [38]. The aim of such a program is to reach a personal transformation of the veterinary medicine students. The curriculum is designed in an interactive way that includes varies different learning formats. The idea is to enhance the existing technical competencies in the medical field with the non-existing non-technical or so-called life skills. They comprise communication, teamwork and professionalism as well as emotional intelligence, leadership, wisdom and creativity [38]. However, do interactive games alone really teach those key competencies? Alternatively, can those leadership programs also be enhanced through different approaches? Leadership programs might be maximized through more intensive incorporation of real-life leaders because they have the potential to inspire managers and future leaders. These positive role models serving as teachers will enhance the quality of training programs and may lead to a new generation of highly motivated leaders [29]. Furthermore, it is important to integrate cross-cultural issues to a greater extent into the leadership training programs because their understanding is crucial for leaders in a global environment. Through this cultural integration, many misunderstandings and cultural barriers can be overcome [29]. This might also very well apply to veterinary practices as veterinarians and veterinary technicians are much more flexible nowadays and relocate easier to other cities and even countries. This can also be seen in the long-running veterinary leadership program of Cornell University that provides a chance for veterinary students from an international background to join a comprehensive leadership and research program [16]. Special leadership programs like the University of Pennsylvania's School of Veterinary Medicine in cooperation with Wharton Executive Education of the University of Pennsylvania focus on an international approach as global health leader programs [37].

Another maximization of leadership programs, especially for female leaders is the change in the program because women require different skills than men. They require less action learning like exploring the Mount Everest but in contrast, more exercises to get out of their purely female role models and to be able to lead in a male-dominated business world.

16.2.3. Critical Aspects of Leadership Programs

"Leadership courses can only teach skills. They can't teach character or vision, and indeed, they don't even try" [12, p.155].

If aspiring managers require excursions to e.g. the Mount Everest region as offered by Wharton School for its MBA students in order to understand what it takes to be a leader [20], then things went fundamentally wrong. If a potential leader does not understand what it takes to be a leader, he will never be one, and he will never become one. Certain skills can be enhanced through the leadership training programs, but the strong will of the individual to lead and to share his vision is something that has to come from deep inside. The word leadership also seems to be too universally used nowadays because real leaders inspire their followers and motivate them to implement their vision. This is not the case in the broad range of so-called leaders because they are just managers [29].

The wide range of partly very expensive leadership programs has opened a new business line for business schools and leadership institutes to attract managers who are hopeful to fulfill their dream to become a leader. It is arguable if those courses are offered in order to improve managerial skills or mainly of making money through creating a leadership hype. However, only certain skills can be taught but character and the personal will and strength is inherited and can never be taught. Therefore, the usefulness of leadership training programs might not be debatable for managers to acquire more skills and enhance their performance, but they will never create leaders if the leadership skill was not already inherited [29].

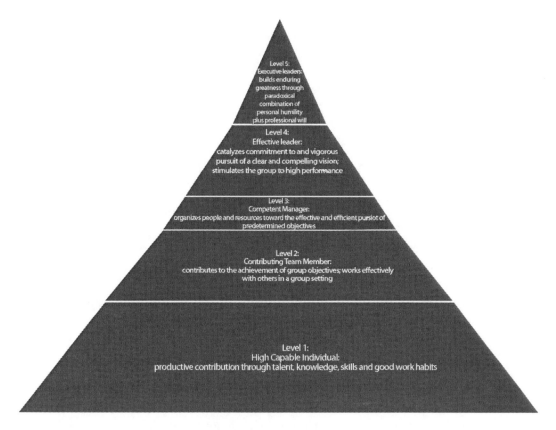

Figure 16.1. Leadership level pyramid [5].

16.3. EMPOWERMENT

Like leadership, the term "Empowerment" has risen to the public interest in the past decades. It has been defined in many ways but taking responsibility and accountability are features that can be found throughout. It is a managerial concept to motivate employees and to make them "buy in" the organizational change. However, fear and resistance might arise among managers because they might fear to lose control. Employees also can resist because they are afraid of being accountable for their work and decisions. Cultural differences might as well lead to non-applicability of empowerment [1].

16.3.1. Definition of Empowerment

What does empowerment really mean? Empowerment has become a major topic in the past two decades due to a wide variety of definitions and meaning. This has led to a lot of misunderstandings, too. Sometimes people believe that empowerment means to let the control go and thus subsequently let subordinates or even projects go out of hand [31]. Empowerment is "an understood authority for employees to act (e.g. make changes), take responsibility, and accept accountability" [33, p.323]. Moreover, it can be defined that "empowering people is giving them knowledge, skills, self-awareness, authority, resources, opportunity and freedom to manage themselves and be accountable for their behavior and performance" [20, p.216]. Two aspects of empowerment can be identified. One is the personal empowerment and the other one the empowerment of the way how we work. The former is the empowerment which gives the individual the feeling of responsibility and empowerment in their lives without circumstances impacting this feeling. The latter has to do with the work atmosphere and environment which we create to enhance self-esteem and growth as well as autonomy in others [1, 31].

16.3.2. Empowerment in Work Places and Veterinary Practices

Leaders should empower their employees to achieve an innovative work environment where employees contribute with their ideas to improve the business. One way to fulfill this aim is to work in teams [33]. Through empowerment, employees will also be enabled to take the necessary steps to implement a vision and the respective goals and objectives [20]. Furthermore, empowerment leads to continuous learning for the leader himself, not only for the employee. Therefore, it can be regarded as a mutual learning process in which the leader learns about his empowered followers, and they learn about their leader. This leads to a kind of interactive learning process [36].

Moreover, empowerment raises self-awareness of the strengths and weaknesses of an individual as well as stimulates the intellect and imagination of the empowered staff. Through delegation of challenging tasks and decision-making authority, employees can be motivated to work actively towards a goal. Opportunities have to be given to the employees to be able to perform well. It is also important in the empowering process to share knowledge and find ways to reward performance as well as learning to motivate the staff further. Coaching and training are inevitable for the empowerment because more skills need to be acquired and developed to fulfill the positions and responsibilities given. However, the empowered employees have to accept the responsibilities given to them and to be self-determined and work autonomously [20]. In order to work effectively, empowerment requires people who are able, confident and who want to take the control [11]. Moreover, empowerment can strengthen the feeling of self-worthiness and self-efficacy of an individual as a benefit of this positive interactive participation. This can be regarded as a part of collective leadership in its positive form [7].

How does empowerment reflect in veterinary practices? Empowerment in this field leads to the situation that the employee starts to own his job due to increased authority and responsibility. On one hand, empowerment results in increased problem-solving, innovation and creativity and on the other hand in a higher number of mistakes initially. Those mistakes can be regarded as an opportunity to improve and to learn. Empowerment also leads to increased productivity through either financial empowerment as veterinary practice owner or partner or emotional empowerment as a motivated employee [2].

Positive points for empowerment are the fact of having important work assignments to do as well as discretion on the job. Moreover, the visibility for the tasks as well as the connection to other staff members and the motivation of subordinates to participate actively in the work are key issues of empowerment [15]. Empowerment through leadership leads to trust among the staff as well as the feeling of integration and belonging of staff to the organization [19]. A main feature of empowerment is the opportunities for employees to take big decisions and the openness of leaders whom their staff can invent new things. This leads in return to freer time and chances top vacations of leaders thus giving them space to think again [6].

Empowerment can be divided into stages e.g. five stages [31]. The first one is the decision-making of the manager. In the second stage, the manager invites suggestions from his team, which are discussed in stage three. Stage four sees a joint decision-making of the management and its team whereas in stage five, the decision-making authority is delegated to the team. This means that the team has reached the autonomy to take even important decisions on their own [31].

Nevertheless, empowerment should not be mistaken with the need for control because it leads to a multiplication of the power. Furthermore, emotional intelligence is a prerequisite for empowerment. Cultural differences as well as different local values have a major impact on empowerment and the extent of a participative leadership style [20].

16.3.3. Advantages and Limitations of Empowerment

Empowering people is usually performed through a participative leadership style. This increases the participation of staff as well as their motivation and work performance. Moreover, the quality of work and productivity increases [20]. Other positive outcomes of empowerment are continuous improvement, better responses to the customers and efficiency which lead to innovation and enhanced customer satisfaction [8].

Another advantage of empowerment is that poor morale, absenteeism and turnover are reduced [17]. Empowerment has the major advantage that not only the employees become more motivated, but also the relationships to their superiors, work process, employees among themselves and the community get changed [11]. Moreover, business organizations with empowerment serve as role models and therefore, can contribute to transfer this model to societies [34].

A positive point for empowerment is the fact that empowerment serves as the prerequisite for organizational change approaches like total quality management and self-managed teams [22].

Limitations of empowerment can be cultural differences, e.g. in the case of high-power distance. Such a high-power distance may lead to employees who do not want to take decisions and responsibilities. Strong individualism can also prove as a limitation to empowerment although individualistic people tend very much to be autonomous, but they are not comfortable in self-managing teams [20].

16.3.4. Difficulties and Problems of Empowerment

Empowerment can only work when the senior management is not tied up in bureaucracy. Other obstacles to empowerment of employees are also when the senior management lacks confidence, self-esteem, trust and leadership [20].

The risk of failure of empowerment has to be taken into consideration as well as the possible abuse of the power given to the employees. It might be also likely that employees are reluctant to take over the responsibilities. Other problems with empowerment are that even managers have to learn more skills in order to empower their employees [20]. Some managers fear to lose control if they empower their employees [9].

Resistance to empower their employees can be frequently found in managers from both, middle-level and senior-level. However, not only managers resist to empowerment, but also non-managerial staff. They are afraid of the responsibilities and that they will be held accountable if something goes wrong [20].

The fear and resistance of employees can be overcome by giving them more time to get used to the idea of empowerment and to implement gradually and to apply it. Moreover, it might also help to enhance trust that all employees have to take on new risks. Training is another vital help to gather support for empowerment. Such a major change in organizational culture requires a transition time and training to enable employees to implement this empowerment concept correctly [30].

Another problem of empowerment is the fact that many organizations are not ready yet due to vertical command chains. This affects especially the middle-level managers which are supposed to be leaders themselves [14]. They form the highest group to resist against empowerment followed by the senior management and junior management. The main reasons of resistance are that the managers are afraid of the new and unwilling to let their power go to their empower subordinates as well as risk aversion [27].

However, the implementation might be difficult, which has led to the fact that empowerment did not really live up to its promise. Through the major focus on empowerment, other equally important psychological mechanisms have been neglected [22].

Further problems of empowerment are the fact that it seems to be more difficult to empower ethnic minorities and women because they do not stick to their responsibilities. This shows clearly that cultural differences hamper empowerment.

Moreover, it is estimated in the United States of America that approximately 20% of employees are afraid of empowerment and another 5% is not able to be integrated in a transformational empowerment system. Employees do not really want to take responsibilities, a fact that is applicable even to developed countries.

These findings lead to major problems of multinational companies and organizations because it might be possible that empowerment works in the subsidiaries in one country. However, in the subsidiary in another country empowerment might simply not work due to cultural barriers and differences [30].

16.4. CONCLUSION

To conclude it seems that leaders are born and the opportunities and experiences in their life have shaped them to the leaders they finally became. The wide range of partly very expensive leadership programs has opened a new business line for business schools and leadership institutes to attract managers who are hopeful about fulfilling their dream to become a leader. It is arguable if those courses are offered in order to improve managerial skills or mainly of making money through creating a leadership hype. However, only certain skills can be taught but the character, and the personal will and strength is inherited and can never be taught. Therefore, the usefulness of leadership training programs for veterinarians might not be debatable for managers to acquire more skills and enhance their performance, but they will never create real leaders if the leadership will and skills were not already inherited.

Empowerment is an important feature for organizational change and reflects a participative leadership style. It has attracted wide-spread interest, and many publications have focused on this topic. Moreover, it has major advantages through staff motivation, which leads to enhanced work quality. In the veterinary world, leadership and empowerment can be used as excellent assets for improved productivity, motivations and thus subsequent increased business. However, this requires strong leaders in the veterinary practice as well as motivated and capable staff members who are ready to take on more responsibilities and challenges.

Leaders are not made. They are born. Managers can be made, but excellent managers have inherited integrity, character and feeling for business and people and have not learnt this knowledge through theories.

REFERENCES

[1]   Abu Aabed, A. (2007). Elective Leadership: Empowerment. Assignment Strathclyde International MBA. University of Strathclyde. Graduate School of Business. Glasgow, UK.

[2]   Ackermann, L. (2007). Blackwell's five minute veterinary practice management consult. Blackwell Publishing. Ames, Iowa.

[3]   Bass, B.M. (1990). From transactional to transformational leadership: learning to share a vision. *Organizational Dynamics*, 18, Winter.

[4]   Bennis, W. (2006). The four competencies of leadership. Chapter 10. http://www.phyton.rice.edu./~arb/Courses/610_06_hew_10.pdf (Accessed on April 8, 2007).

[5]   Bock, W. (2007). Are leaders born or made? httw://interpret.co.za/html/art/ are_leaders_born_or_made_.php (Accessed on April 8, 2007).

[6]   Boorstin, J. (2003). How the best leaders empower people. Executive Leader. Vol. 18, no. 11, November. http://leadershipthatlasts.com/archives/12-17-03.htm (Accessed on April 8, 2007).

[7]   Burns, J.M. (1998). Empowerment for change. Rethinking Leadership Working Papers. Academy of Leadership Press. http://www.academy.umd.edu/ publications/klspdocs/ jburns_p1.htm (Accessed on April 8, 2007).

[8]   Bushe, G.R., Havlovic, S.J. and Croetzer, G. (1996). Exploring empowerment from the inside out. *Journal for Quality and Participation,* 19 (2). pp. 36-45.

[9]   Capozzoli, T.K. (1995). Managers and leaders: a matter of cognitive difference. *Journal of Leadership Studies,* 2 (3). pp. 20-29.

[10]   Chadwick, M.J. (2007). Leaders are born – and made. http://www.rec.org/REC/ programs/EMTC/insight/vol31/interview.html (Accessed on April 8, 2007).

[11]   Ciulla, J.B. (1996). Leadership and the problem of bogus empowerment. Ethics and Leadership Working Papers. Academy of Leadership Press. http://www.academy.umd.edu/publications/klspdocs/jciul_p1.htm (Accessed on April 8, 2007).

[12]   Chakraborty, S.K. (1995). *Ethics in management: Vedic Perspective.* Dehli, Oxford University Press.

[13]   Collins, J. (2005). Level 5 Leadership. The triumph of humility and fierce resolve. Best of HBR 2001. The high performance organization. July –August 2005. Harvard Business Review. http://www.hbr.org/hb-main/resources/pdfs/comm/microsoft/level-five.pdf (Accessed on January 14th, 2011).

[14]   Colvin, R.E. (2001). Leading from the middle: a challenge for middle managers. Paper presented at the Bernhard M.Brass Festschrift, State University of New York at Binghamton, May 31-June 1.

[15]   Conger, J.A. (1992). Learning to lead: the art of transforming managers into leaders. 1st ed. Jossey-Bass Inc. Publishers. San Francisco, California.

[16]   Cornell University (2009). Leadersgip program for veterinary students, 20th anniversary issue, 2009. http://www.vet.cornell.edu/oge/Leadership/docs/report090909.pdf (Accesssed on January 18th, 2011).

[17]   Densison, D. (1984). Bringing corporate culture to the bottom line. *Organizational Dynamics,* 13 (2). pp. 4-22.

[18]   Dixon, N. (1985). Why lefties make the best leaders. *Personnel Management.* November, pp. 36-39.

[19]   Ford, J.M. (1998). Some common sense about leadership. Vantage press, New York.

[20]   Gill, R. (2006). Theory and practice of leadership. Sage Publications. London, Thousand Oaks, Delhi.

[21]   Graf, J. (2004). Leaders are born, not made…and other popular myths. JPT, April. http://www.spe.org/spe/jpt/jsp/jptmonthlysection/o,2440,1104_11038_2354946_23679 (Accessed on April 8, 2007).

[22]   Howard, A. (1997). High involvement leadership: moving from talk to action. *Empowerment in Organizations,* Vol. 5 Iss: 4, pp.185 - 192.

[23]   Hill, L. A. (2004). New manager development for the 21st century. *Academy of Management Executive.* August. p. 122.

[24]   Huth, A.J. (2006). Born to lead or made to manage – We need both http://www.abadvisors.com/pdf/BornToLead.pdf (Accessed on April 8, 2007).

[25]   Johnson, A.M., Vernon, P.A., McCarthy, J.M., Molson, M., Harris, J.A. and Jang, K.L.(1998). Nature vs nurture: are leaders born or made? A behavioral genetic investigation of leadership style. *Twin Research,* dec; 1(4). pp. 216-223.

[26]   Lenz, R.T. (1993). Strategic management and organizational learning: a meta-theory of executive leadership. In: J. Hendry, G. Johnson and J. Newton (eds), *Strategic thinking: Leadership and the management of change.* Chichester: John Wiley&Sons.

[27] Lowe, P. (1994). Empowerment: management dilemma, leadership challenge. *Executive Development,* 7 (1), pp. 10-21.

[28] Maltby, D.E. (2007). The state of leadership theory and training today. http://www.biola.edu/academics/scs/leadership/resoruces/bornormade/ (Accessed on April 8, 2007).

[29] Müller, M.G. (2007). Elective Leadership: Are leaders born or made?Assignment Strathclyde International MBA. University of Strathclyde. Graduate School of Business. Glasgow, UK.

[30] Offermann, L.R. (1997). Leading and empowering diverse followers. The Balance of Leadership & Followership Working Papers. Academy of Leadership Press. http://www.academy.umd.edu/publications/klspdocs/loffe_p1.htm (Accessed on April 8, 2007).

[31] Pastor, J. (1996). Empowerment: what it is and what it is not. Empowerment in Organizations. Vol. 4, No. 2, pp. 5-7.http://www.leader-values.com/Content/detail Print.asp?ContentDetailID=86 (Accessed on April 8, 2007).

[32] Powell, S.R. (2007). The power of positive peer influence: leadership training for today's teens. Princeton Center for Leadership Training. http://www.princetonleadership.org/pgc-art1.pdf (Accessed on April 8, 2007).

[33] Smith, G.P. (1997). The new leader. *Bringing creativity and innovation to the workplace.* St. Lucie Press, Florida, USA.

[34] Spreitzer, G. (2007). Giving peace a chance: Organizational leadership, empowerment, and peace. *J.Organiz.Behav.*28, pp.1077-1095.DOI:10.1002/job.487.

[35] Tracy, B. (2007). Leaders are born, not made. Brian Tracy Articles. http://www.briantracyarticles.com/business/Leaders-Are-Made-Not-Born.html (Accessed on April 8, 2007).

[36] Vaill, P.B. (1997). The learning challenges of leadership. The Balance of Leadership & Followership Working Papers. Academy of Leadership Press. http://www.academy.umd.edu/publications/klspdocs/pvaill_p1.htm (Accessed on April 8, 2007).

[37] Wharton University of Pennsylvania (2011). Penn executive veterinary leadership program: making an impact as a global health leader. http://executiveeducation.wharton.upenn.edu/open-enrollment/leadership-development-programs/executive-veterinary-leadership.cfm (Accessed on January 18th, 2011).

[38] Washington State University (2011). AVMAVeterinary Leadership experience. http://www.vetmed.wsu.edu/orgVLE/rationale.aspx (Accessed on January 18th, 2011).

Chapter 17

PERFORMANCE MANAGEMENT

ABSTRACT

Performance management systems are a common feature in the modern business world. The advantages and disadvantages of the respective performance management systems are discussed in detail under special consideration of veterinary businesses. Despite their advantages and disadvantages, they start to enter the veterinary business world especially in large veterinary hospitals and veterinary medicine universities. This chapter discusses the different models and their applicability in veterinary practices. A special balanced scorecard and performance prism has been developed as tailor-made approaches for veterinary performance measurements for even small veterinary practices.

17.1. INTRODUCTION

The search for excellence was not a common widespread feature of the business world before the 1980s [13]. This changed dramatically after the first main book on excellence in business was published in 1982 [24]. Over the years, plenty of attempts have been made in order to try to find the secret of companies performing with excellence and outperforming their competitors. However, despite many improvements and introduction of new theories and approaches to define performance excellence, there is still no final answer to this question [13]. Although originating from the business world, the desire and need for increased productivity and performance as well as reduced costs in a more and more competitive world has found its way into the healthcare sector as well. Attempts to introduce benchmarking and productivity measures in hospitals have been made e.g. in Canada and Finland [7, 16] and in the veterinary university field [1, 6].

17.2. VETERINARY PERFORMANCE MANAGEMENT

High performance in jobs and their redesign is a vital driver of performance management as well as productivity [18]. Four different areas can contribute to enhanced job performance: span of control, span of accountability, span of influence and span of support. By widening or reducing any of these spans, a different job output is the result thus enhancing the staff performance [29]. Popular concepts of performance management are the Balanced Scorecard (BSC) or Performance Prism.

17.2.1. Balanced Scorecard

The concept of the "balanced scorecard" (BSC) is a strategic measurement and performance management system, which includes a wide range of performance indicators [3] and is regarded as a more holistic approach towards performance management [26]. However, its main focus lies on the financial aspect of organizations [9]. The BSC is a strategic model integrating the organization's vision and strategy into a well-focused implementation with four perspectives: financial perspective, customer perspective, business process perspective and growth and learning perspective. All those perspectives are monitored and scored by the objectives, targets, measures and initiatives [9, 20].

The customer perspective is about information of how the customer regards the company and has been recently regarded as customer resource management [26]. Apart from normal customer view measures, the BSC provides the possibility to measure customer profitability through parameters like "percentage of unprofitable customers," or "dollars lost in unprofitable customer relationships" [12, p.2].

The financial perspective gives information about the shareholders view of the company whereas the internal business perspective looks at the core competencies and ways to excel in order to reach a competitive advantage. Innovation, growth and learning are the fourth important perspective that is tied directly to the value of the company [26]. However, the integration of the community has been missing, which has been suggested as fifth perspective [23].

However, when developing a BSC, great care needs to be taken about the right understanding and process of developing as otherwise the outcome of the newly developed BSC might not be as desired and useful [27]. Therefore, the intention of the BSC to balance the main perspectives often fails in practice thus leading to unbalanced or biased scorecards in many companies [20]. One of the reasons for these unbalanced scorecards is the fact that the design of the BSC mainly focuses on the key success drivers of the companies [14]. Finally, the balanced scorecard can only succeed through proper implementation and organizational leadership [20, 26].

17.2.1.1. Balanced Scorecard in Veterinary Practice

Despite being developed as a business model, the BSC has recently found its way into the performance management of hospitals [4, 25, 30]. Several benefits of a good BSC for the healthcare sector have been identified as being customer insight, refocusing of internal operations, strengthening of customer acquisition efforts and relations, increase of loyalty and return on value as well as attracting internal stakeholders [17]. However, being different from normal businesses, the perspectives of a hospital balanced scorecard needs to be adjusted. Research [25, 30] suggests four perspectives being clinical utilization and outcomes, system integration and change, financial performance and condition as well as patient and family satisfaction for the Canadian hospital complex continuing care. A balanced performance measurement for hospitals also includes information about health outcomes apart from productivity indicators [8].

Measurement of performance can be done with the very popular Balanced Scorecard, which has been so far mainly implemented in large hospitals, and those affiliated with teaching [4]. Lately, the BSC has found its way in the veterinary university world as a complete performance planning process has been drafted at the Iowa State University [6].

Table 17.1. Sample Balanced Scorecard for the veterinary practice [20]

Financial and Social Cost		Customers	
Goals	Measures	Goals	Measures
Sustainability	Cash flow	Waiting time	Per minutes
	Sales growth	Complaints	Number of complaints per time
Success	Increase of services	Response to questions	Time, friendliness, proficiency
Profit	Increased income	Service value ration	Number of requested services
Internal Processes		Innovation and Learning	
Goals	Measures	Goals	Measures
Capability	Service quality	New techniques	Successful application
New services introduction	Actual information schedule vs. plan	Service focus	Percentage of services equal to X% of income
Efficiency	Productivity per staff	Staff learning	New skills
Service excellence	Time, cost, number of mistakes, number of complaints		

A more sophisticated approach to performance management by using the Balanced Scorecard can be done in larger veterinary practices or hospitals. The BSC can be used for different time frames like monthly, quarterly or yearly depending on the different KPI's. The BCS can cover various divisions like the overall group, the management and administration, R&D, marketing and the manufacturing and sales department. One of the veterinary practices' main competitive advantages should be the strongly skilled, motivated and loyal employee force. Therefore special KPI's measure their performance and satisfaction.

17.2.1.2. Advantages from Introducing Reports Based on BSC Approach

Reports using the Balanced Scorecard approachlead to meaningful results that provide valuable information about the company. Moreover, such reports create an enhanced communication among all levels in the organization and con-currency of the organization. Another benefit is the understanding of cause and effect relationships that can only be assumed otherwise. Equally important, the BSC reports lead to a perfect fit between the strategy and mission of the organization and its core competencies as well as the environmental influences. They help as test environment for a strategic hypothesis and establish the accounting for organizational and topic interdependency [23].

Even the best strategy fails, if badly executed, which represent one of the major reasons for strategy failures. This problem can be overcome by shifting from traditional financial-oriented performance measures like budgets or shareholder values to a complete performance management program [11]. Over the past years, the BSC has matured from a performance measures system into a comprehensive management system, the so-called strategy focused organization (SFO). Its predominant challenges are the sustainability of the efforts because it is a wider step than just to work with a well-developed Balanced Scorecard [10]. The strategy-focused organization is based on five main principles.

Table 17.2. BSC for larger veterinary practices and hospitals:
Financial perspective [20]

Practice Division	Financial Perspective	
	Goals	Measures (KPIs)
Overall / Management	High turnover	Increase in turnover compared to previous year's turnover
	High net profit	Increase in net profit compared to previous year's turnover
	High total profit	Increase in total profit compared to previous year's turnover
	High divisional income	Income of division/ department in US $ / number of staff
	High cash flow	Cash flow compared to last year's cash flow
	Revenue growth	Increase in revenue /operating costs
	Expense to revenue ratio	Number of expenses / number of revenue
	High share price	Increase in share price compared to previous year's share price
	Reduced costs	Number of total costs / number of operating costs
Innovation	High new product/service value	High profitability / new product or service
	Low innovation costs	Low innovation costs / newly developed product or service
Marketing	Revenue growth	Increase in revenue / operating cost
	Attraction of new customer market	Number of new customers per marketing costs
	Gross margins	Increase in gross margin compared to previous year's gross margins
Sales	Sales growth	Increase in sales per product
	Sales force productivity	Spending in US $ / direct staff costs + indirect staff costs + overhead costs
	Sales cost	Sales cost per revenue in %

Table 17.3. BSC for larger veterinary practices and hospitals:
Customer perspective [20]

Practice Division	Customer Perspective	
	Goals	Measures
Overall / Management	Increase in market share	Increase in market share compared to the previous year's market share
	Brand image	Number of special requested products

Practice Division	Customer Perspective	
	Goals	Measures
	Waiting time	Waiting time in hours/days until service gets delivered
Innovation	New customer market	New innovative services per new customer market
Marketing	Number of new customers	Number of new customers per service
Sales	Customer satisfaction	Number of complaints / number of sold products
	Loyal customer base	Number of re-orders / customer per time period
	Customer number	Number of daily customers / total staff
	Customer profitability	Percentage of unprofitable customers per total customer number
	Customer unprofitability	US $ lost in unprofitable customer relationships
	Customer staff ratio	Number of daily served customers / individual staff

Table 17.4. BSC for larger veterinary practices and hospitals:
Internal business perspective [20]

Practice Division	Internal Business Perspective	
	Goals	Measures
Overall / Management	Forecast accuracy	Number of wrong forecasts / forecasting period
	Employment security for staff	Number of lay-offs per division
	Employees satisfaction	Number of resignations / division or department
	Productivity per staff	Number of performed services per staff
	Mistake rate	Number of mistakes / service
	Long-terms relations with suppliers	Number of replaced suppliers / time period
	Order fulfillment speed	Time to fulfill order / number of orders
Innovation	High new service development	Number of new innovative ideas / number of realized new services
Marketing	Innovative marketing campaigns	Number of new customers / number of product campaigns
Sales	Staff sales ratio	Number of transactions / direct staff costs
		Number of sales / staff
	Sales time ratio	Number of sales / time
	Sales staff knowledge	Number of unanswered customer questions / staff

The first one is the mobilization of change through executive leadership, which helps for governance and strategic development. The leaders have to develop a sense of urgency of understanding change and to create leadership teams, including executive teams and professional specialists from different departments. Moreover, this leadership team needs to develop the vision and strategy for the company. Through BSC, reports provide decision-makers and leadership team with the advantage to rely on profound and up-to-date data for aligning strategies [11].

Table 17.5. BSC for larger veterinary practices and hospitals:
Innovation, Growth, Learning perspective [20]

Practice Division	Innovation, Growth, Learning Perspective	
	Goals	Measures
Overall / Management	New skills for staff	Number of new skill certifications / number of staff
	Staff training	Number of training/ number of staff
	Latest IT technology	Number of time saving / number of new IT technology
	Center of excellence through certifications	Number of latest certifications e.g. ISO or CPD / services
	Advanced equipments	Number of advanced equipments / number of total equipments
Innovation	Cost-efficiency	Savings in time and $ / innovative idea
Marketing	Marketing training	Number of new marketing skills / number of staff
Sales	Introduction of new products	Number of new products / number of income through new products

The second pillar is the translating of strategy into operating terms through strategic maps and the BSC. The Balanced Scorecard reports can be of great benefit for the defining of KPIs and success factors on a short-term productivity oriented and long-term growth-oriented basis [11]. The third element of the SFO that represents the alignment of the organization with the strategy can be helped through the BSC. The BSC has the great advantage and power to describe and measure the strategy of the single organization's departments. It is the task of the BSC to coordinate and link the different departmental functions and strategies to a comprehensive framework for the whole organization. This will lead to synergies among support and business units to fit in their corporate role [11]. The fourth part of the SFO is the integration of every staff in the organization to understand fully the strategy through communication and education. Everybody in the organization needs to be personally aligned with it through their individual objectives in the BSC. The execution of strategy and enhanced performance can be linked with balanced pay cheques or incentives to the fulfilled targets of the BSC which poses another major advantage of the BSC reporting system [11]. The last pillar of the SFO is the change to make strategy formulation a continual process. The Balanced Scorecard can be used very well to link the strategy to the budgeting process. The complete BSC financial and non-financial reports are discussed on a regular, e.g. quarterly basis to review the achievement and to correct non-alignments. Furthermore, the BSC paves the way for further strategy development through strategic learning [11].

17.2.2. Performance Prism

However, despite the popularity of the BSC, it is derived from strategy and lacks the emphasis on all its stakeholders, esp. suppliers and employees [21] as well as regulators, local community, intermediaries and pressure groups [22]. In order to achieve a more stakeholder oriented performance measure model, a five-faceted model, the so-called Performance Prism (PP), was developed considering the stakeholder satisfaction, stakeholder contribution as well as strategies, processes and capabilities [21].

The PP focuses in the first place on the stakeholder. However, this is not a unilateral approach as not only the satisfaction of the stakeholder counts, but also their contribution to the business company thus being a unique feature among all different performance management models [22]. This model can be flexibly adjusted to the individual business and enhances the thinking process of all concerned parties [22]. It provides also a framework for dealing with a difficult business situation, e.g. a recession [2].This model seems to fit the veterinary practice in a much better way as the customer or client always comes first.

The Performance Prism focuses in the first place on the stakeholders which are the pet owners, practice staff, suppliers, community, animal rescue groups, etc.. However, it is not a unilateral approach, which takes only the satisfaction of those stakeholders into consideration. In contrast, those stakeholders also have to contribute to the veterinary practice thus being a unique feature among all different performance management models [22]. This performance management model can be flexibly adjusted consequently making it ideal for the individual veterinary practice. It provides also a framework for dealing with difficult business situations, e.g. a recession [2].

Table 17.6. Performance prism measures for the veterinary practice [20]

Stakeholder Satisfaction	Strategy	Process	Capability	Stakeholder Contribution	Financial Performance
Waiting time for pet owners	High quality services	Introduction of new services	Staff training, CPD	Staff knowledge + experience	Increase of income
Number of requested services	Cost efficiency	Introduction of new products	Advanced equipment	Loyalty and trust by pet owners	Increase of services
Number of complaints	Excellent reputation of practice	Cost of services	Facility suitable for services	High reputation by suppliers + clients	Increase of product sale
Number of revisits	Quality care with certifications	Productivity per staff	Additional services like laboratory	Info about new equipment by suppliers	Increase of cash flow
Employment security for staff	Long-terms relations with stakeholders	Number of mistakes	Latest IT technology	Word-by-mouth advertisement by pet owners	Reduced costs

17.3. VETERINARY PRODUCTIVITY MEASURES

In the service sector, it is more difficult to measure productivity and to increase it [19]. The measurement of productivity rates in the hospital environment is useful but needs to be adjusted and expanded [28].

17.3.1. Common Veterinary Productivity Measures

Usually, the common measure for hospital productivity is the "cost per patient day." This does not include the outpatients thus leading to a too low productivity of the hospital [16]. Another common productivity measure, the number of admissions or out-patient visits was unsuitable for hospitals [8]. In the veterinary field, the average revenue from specialty transactions, all other sources and practice have been used as productivity measures [1]. Moreover, the average productivity per staff has been measured by the FTE (full-time equivalent time equivalent) [1] although FTE is not regarded as sufficient and useful for hospital environment [28].

Alternative indicators have to be introduced considering the internal operations and external hospital business environment leading to an expansion of common productivity measures [28]. Specifying benchmarking for hospitals with introducing multiple productivity and performance measures is supposed to tackle the special hospital environment [8] and to describe output of hospitals better [15].

One way of correcting the hospital productivity measures is the separation of outpatient costs and services from inpatient costs and services [16]. New measurement units for output of hospitals have been introduced like the so-called "care episode" being the number of admissions and outpatient visits for a patient due to the same disease [7]. This can be measured by the newly developed "episode productivity" as well as the average number of admissions or costs per episode [7, 8]. However, this might not be completely applicable to veterinary medicine as much of the aftercare depends on the correct husbandry procedures of the owner.

Another useful step can be to sort the most significant patient groups according to their economic impact and to identify the possibility of saving costs and resources in these groups [8]. This approach for productivity benchmarks is also called "diagnosis-related groups" which helps to standardize the mixed patient clientele [15]. Apart from these diagnoses-related groups, other productivity measures can be formed according to specialties and wards [15].

Labor costs of hospital staff like nursing staff can be reduced by introducing productivity measures without reducing patient care [5]. In a hospital environment, the productivity measures have to be differentiated according to departments like administration and finance and technical staff e.g. nurses. In order to establish productivity measures in the nursing department, the work processes and standards have to be defined and analyzed. This is achieved by breaking down tasks like patient-care hours and benchmarking, which translate into the budget and staffing plans. However, certain "staffing exceptions" need to be integrated with great flexibility in the productivity measures for special circumstances [5].

17.3.2. Key Performance Indicators in Veterinary Practice

Regarding the main KPIs in the veterinary practice, a differentiation can be taken between out-patient practice and hospitalized pets. Different productivity measures have to be put in place in the medical, laboratory and administrative area.

Out-Patient Clinic
In the out-patient practice, the productivity measures have to be divided into the pet owner-oriented KPIs and staff-related KPIs. Pet owner-related productivity parameters are customer satisfaction, number of complaints, re-visits, waiting time, information on the phone about medical issues. This can be translated into the following KPIs:

- Number of complaints / number of visits
- Waiting time in minutes until a pet enters consultation room
- Number of daily pet owners / total staff
- Number of treated out-patients pets / individual staff
- Number of re-visits / pet owner
- Income of out-patient visit / direct staff costs + indirect staff costs + consumables + overhead costs

In-Patient Clinic
The hospitalized pets can be split according to diagnosis profiles for short-term hospitalization (1-7 days) which poses the majority of cases in the general small animal practice, medium-terms stays (8-21 days) and long-terms stays (> 21 days).

For each hospitalization period, the following KPIs can be measured:

- Number of treated hospitalized pets for short / medium / long-term hospitalization / individual staff
- Number of surgeries / day
- Number of surgeries / individual staff
- Number of disease's recurrences / care episode
- Income of an in-patient for short / medium / long-term hospitalization/ direct staff costs + indirect staff costs + consumables + overhead costs

Administration Productivity Measures
- Number of transactions / direct staff costs
- Number of transactions / time
- Saving on the cost / budget
- Number of transactions / number of staff

Laboratory Productivity Measures
- Income of outside samples / direct staff costs + indirect staff costs + consumables + overhead costs

- Income of hospital samples / direct staff costs + indirect staff costs + consumables + overhead costs
- Income of laboratory department/ number of staff
- Number of samples performed per day / individual staff
- Number of samples / number of quality controls

17.4. INTRODUCTION OF TAILOR-MADE PERFORMANCE MANAGEMENT SYSTEM FOR THE VETERINARY PRACTICE

The Balanced Scorecard system ties the business strategy with the performance management model to reach a comprehensive approach. This can be helpful not only in profit-oriented businesses, government organizations or hospitals, but might be a suitable approach for a veterinary hospital as well.

A major point is the influence of stakeholders on the veterinary practice's business being internal or external stakeholders. As the BSC does not consider the contribution of the stakeholders, this is an important feature which needs to be added to the PMS.

17.4.1. PMS Components

Having so far no performance management system is in place, a specialized combined performance management model with features of the BSC and PP for the veterinary practice needs to be developed. This approach considers:

- Stakeholder satisfaction
- Stakeholder contribution
- Practice strategy
- Processes
- Capabilities
- Financial performance

Stakeholder Satisfaction
When talking about stakeholders, it is essential to define who internal and external stakeholders are. Moreover, mere satisfaction might not be enough for a long-term relationship as it might be desirable to reach a high satisfaction level of all stakeholders.

The internal stakeholders of the veterinary practice are:

- Employees
- Support staff

Employees and support staff want a safe and secure workplace with good salary and to be recognized for their work.

The external stakeholders of the veterinary practice are:

- Customers for veterinary services
- Customers for other services, e.g. nutritional advice, grooming, puppy parties
- Customers for laboratory services
- Suppliers
- Special pet communities
- Others

Their satisfaction comes from a variety of different issues like quality excellence, reasonable pricing, correct and repeated orders, timely payment, as well as fast and accurate services.

Stakeholder Contribution

Stakeholders can contribute in a manifold way to the business process. They can give ideas for improvement or process change, their professional experience and knowledge, commitment and loyalty to their work and workplace, trust, support and enhance the recognition and reputation of the business.

Veterinary Practice Strategy

The goals and objectives of the veterinary practice have to be clearly defined. The strategic goals are usually to provide high quality standard treatment of pets and to be a center of excellence. Its objectives are:

- To be a leading veterinary institution
- To have comprehensive business-oriented management approach
- To work cost-efficient

The stakeholders are not explicitly mentioned. However, as being a service institution it is understood that the customer satisfaction should be achieved through the goal of a center of excellence. Moreover, only with a high customer satisfaction, a long-term relationship between the veterinary practice and its clients can be built.

Processes

The general main processes of the veterinary practices should have been mapped. However, new innovative and income generating services have to be developed with close orientation at the customers wishes and requirements. This could be a step away from the core business, but could provide an answer to new customer demands and open up brand new business areas. However, such new services and products have to be introduced in a sustainable way in order not to interfere with the core business, the veterinary treatment.

Capabilities

The facet of capabilities includes the people, practice, technology and infrastructure [22]. This means for the veterinary practices to review the capabilities not only in the medical sector, but also in the administration and laboratory. It includes an advanced IT and technological infrastructure to speed up the processes which need to be applied by the staff.

Financial Performance

The financial performance is another important pillar for the PMS. It includes the sales growth, cash flow and increased income through a higher number of services or new products.

17.4.2. Veterinary Practices PMS Model

For the development of a tailor-made PMS for the veterinary practice, a brainstorming approach can be started with consideration of the major performance points and measures.

Key questions are important issues as they lead to the performance measures.

- What can the veterinary practice introduce to reach high customer satisfaction?
- How can the veterinary practice increase productivity?
- What are the measures of improving the processes?
- How can the veterinary practice increase the income?
- What are the factors involved in reducing the cost?
- What is the strategy of veterinary practice?
- Who are the stakeholders in veterinary practice?
- What is the way to increase the capability of the veterinary practice staff?

It will be useful to design a performance measure sheet with KPIs for the different measures before starting the implementation process, but this might be too far-reaching for the average veterinary practice.

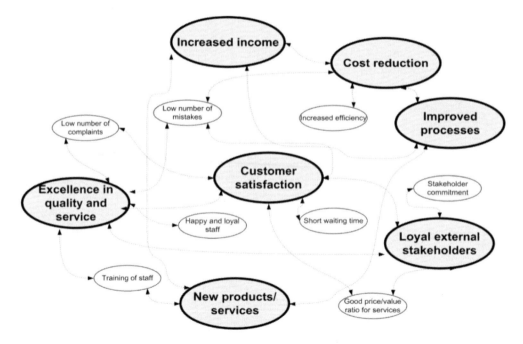

Figure 17.7. Brainstorming model for PMS measures [20].

Table 17.8. Performance measures for the easy tailor-made PMS for the veterinary practice [20]

Stakeholder Satisfaction	Strategy	Process	Capability	Stakeholder Contribution	Financial Performance
Employment security for staff	High quality work	Introduction of new products	Staff training	Staff knowledge + experience	Sales growth
Waiting time	Cost-efficiency	Introduction of new services	Advanced machines	Loyalty and trust	Increase of services
Number of complaints	Extended positive profile	Productivity per staff	Facility extension	High reputation by suppliers + clients	Increase of income
Number of requested services	Center of excellence through accreditations	Cost of services	New skills for staff	Information about new machines by suppliers	Increase of cash flow
Number of revisits	Long-terms relations with stakeholders	Number of mistakes	Latest IT technology	Funding from sponsors	Reduced costs

17.5. CONCLUSION

Performance management systems can be integrated in veterinary practices to identify good and weak business areas and to find ways for improvement. However, the commonly used performance management systems like Balanced Scorecard and Performance Prism are not very useful for introduction in the veterinary world.

They need to be carefully revised and tailor-made for the special needs and requirements of veterinary practices. If this is taken into consideration, such specially designed performance management systems can provide much interesting information for the veterinary practice owner or practice manager. They can then be used to introduce corrective measures that will lead to enhanced business success.

Performance needs to be measured even in the difficult field of veterinary business. Nevertheless, such performance management systems should be kept easy to perform with the absolute minimum of key performance indicators.

For this reason, key performance indicators should be chosen well in order to produce results that are really required. The idea of performance management systems is *not* to increase bureaucracy in the veterinary practice and to overload the staff with computer sheets and paperwork. The veterinary performance management system shall aim to produce relevant reproducible statistical data that can be used to manage the veterinary practice more effectively and efficiently. This leads to increased work volume and customer satisfaction as well as a reduction of mistakes and subsequently maximization of business profits.

REFERENCES

[1]   AAHA (2006). 2005 specialty & referral veterinary practice benchmark study. *American Animal Hospital Association.* http://www.aahanet.org/About_aaha/ Specialty_Benchmrk_Study.pdf (Accessed on June 24th, 2006).

[2]   Adams, C. and Neely, A. (2001). Managing with measures in a downturn. http://www.som.cranfield.ac.uk/som/research/centres/cbp/products/prism.asp (Accessed on July, 2nd, 2006).

[3]   Beech, N., Cairns, G., Livingstone, H., Lockyer, C. and Tsoukas, H. (2005). Performance Management. In: Beech, N., Cairns, G., Livingstone, H., Lockyer, C. and H. Tsoukas. *Managing people in organisations,* Vol. 2. 2nd ed. Glasgow: The Graduate School of Business University of Strathclyde. pp. 384-402.

[4]   Chan Y.-Ch. L. and. Ho, S.-J. K (1997). The use of balanced scorecard in Canadian hospitals. http:// aaahq.org/northeast/2000/q17.pdf (Accessed on September 25th, 2006).

[5]   Garcia, L. (2001). Using productivity measures to control labor costs. Advance for Healthcare Information Executives. February, Vol.5, No.2. http://api-wi.com/checksource.asp?source=articles&pr.72441 (Accessed on June 22nd, 2006).

[6]   Iowa State University (2006). College of Veterinary Medicine Planning and Performance Process. http://www.vetmed.iastate.edu/about/accreditation/ planning_ process .asp (Accessed on June, 21st, 2006).

[7]   Järvelin, J., Linna, M. and Häkkinen, U. (2003). The hospital benchmarking project: productivity information for hospital comparison. Dialogi in English. p. 26. http://www2.stakes.fi/dialogi/english/2003/26.htm (Accessed on June 24th, 2006).

[8]   Junnila, M., Järvelin, J., Linna, M. and Idänpään-Heikkilä, U. (2004). Benchmarking hospital care. Reproduced as licensed to ISQua. http://www.isqua.org.au/ isquaPages /Conferences/amsterdam/AmsterdamWebFiles/webfiles/IND19-10-4/INDPosterAbstracts/Abstracts/IND%20050-doc.pdf.

[9]   Kaplan, R. and Norton, D. (1996). The balanced Scorecard: Translating strategy into action. Cambridge, MA: Harvard Business School Press.

[10]   Kaplan, R. and. Norton, D. (2000). The strategy-focused organisation. October 23. Harvard Business School. Working knowledge for business leaders. http://hbswk.hbs.edu/cgi-bin/print (Accessed on January 27th, 2007).

[11]   Kaplan, R. and Norton, D. (2001). Building a strategy-focused organisation. Reprint #9BO1TCO3. *Ivey Business Journal.* May/June.

[12]   Kaplan, R. (2005). A balanced scorecard approach to measure customer profitability. August 8. Harvard Business School. *Working knowledge for business leaders.* http://hbswk.edu/item/4968.html (Accessed on January 21st, 2007).

[13]   Kirby, D. and Watson, A. (1999). Franchising as a small business development strategy: a qualitative study of operational and 'failed' franchisors in the UK. *Journal of Small Business Enterprise Development,* Vol. 6, No. 4. pp. 314-349.

[14] Leahy, T. (2000). Tailoring the balanced scorecard. Business Finance. August. http://www.businessfinancemag.com/magazines/archives/article.html?articleID=13607 (Accessed on June 21st 2006).

[15] Linna, M. (2006). Benchmarking hospital productivity. Health Policy Monitor. Survey No. 7. http://www.healthpolicymonitor.org/en/About_Us/ Partner_Institutions/ STAKES/Benchmarking_hospital_productivity.html(Accessed on June 24th, 2006).

[16] MacLean, M.B. and Mix, P. (1991). Measuring hospital productivity and output: the omission of outpatient services. *Health Rep.* Vol. 3(3), pp. 229-244.

[17] MacStravic, S. (1999). A really balanced scorecard. *Health Forum Journal* 42, no. 3. pp. 64-67.

[18] McMillan, R. and Mullen, T. (2005a). *Operations management.* Volume 1. 3rd ed. Glasgow: The Graduate School of Business University of Strathclyde.

[19] McMillan, R. and Mullen, T. (2005b). *Operations management.* Volume 2. 3rd ed. Glasgow: The Graduate School of Business University of Strathclyde.

[20] Muller, M.G. (2007). Financial and management accounting. MBA Assignment.University of Strathclyde. *Graduate School of Business.* Glasgow, UK.

[21] Neely, A. and Adams, C. (2000). Perspectives on performance: The Performance Prism. Cranfield School of Management. http://www.som.cranfield.ac.uk/som/research/ centres/cbp/products/prism.asp (Accessed on July, 2nd, 2006).

[22] Neely, A., Adams, C. and Crowe, P. (2006). The Performance Prism in practice. http://www.som.cranfield.ac.uk/som/research/centres/cbp/products/prism.asp (Accessed on July, 2nd, 2006).

[23] Niven, P. (2007). Examining the endurance of the balanced scorecard. http://www.balancedscorecard.biz/articles/examining_endurance_BSC.html (Accessed on January 20th, 2007).

[24] Peters, T. and Waterman, R.H. (2004). In search of excellence. 2nd.ed. *Profile Books.* London.UK.

[25] Pink G.H., McKillopm I., Schraam E.G., Peyram C., Montgomery C. and Baker, G.R.(1997). Creating a balanced scorecard for a hospital system. *J. Health Care Finance.* Fall; 24(1). pp. 55-58.

[26] Scherer, D. (2002). Balanced scorecard overview. Core paradigm. http://www.coreparadigm.com/articles/balancedScorecard.pdf (Accessed on August 29th, 2011).

[27] Schneidermann, A.M. (2004). The balanced scorecard: an approach for linking strategy to action. Http://www.schneidermann.com/the Art_of_PM/what_is_ the_BSC? what_is_the_SC.htm (Accessed on June 21st, 2006).

[28] Serway, G.D., Strum, D.W. and Haug, W.F. (1987). Alternative indicators for measuring hospital productivity. *Hospital Health Service Administration,* August, Vol 32(3). pp. 379-398.

[29] Simons, R. (2005). Designing high performance jobs. *Harvard Business Review.* July-August. pp. 55-62.

[30] Teare, G.F., Baker, G.R., Daniel, I., Hirdes, J.P., Markel, F., McKillop, I., Pink, G.H., Taylor, N., van Maris, B. and Brown, A. (2002). A balanced scorecard for complex care. Reproduced as licensed to ISOQua http://www.isqua.org.au/isquaPages/ Conferences/ paris/ParisAbstractsSlides/Thursday/B08/Abspdf/419%20-%20Teare.pdf

Chapter 18

OCCUPATIONAL HEALTH AND SAFETY MANAGEMENT

ABSTRACT

Health and safety management is becoming more and more important in modern veterinary practice management. It includes a variety of topics like environmental pollution, occupational health and safety, personal injuries, fatalities and property damages. Furthermore, zoonotic diseases of non parasitic and parasitic have to be taken into consideration. In cases of health and safety problems, financial and legal liabilities may arise for the veterinary practice. It is therefore highly important to establish a sound health and safety framework for the practice taking into consideration those issues. Check lists may help to get an overview about the status of the occupational health and safety issues in the veterinary practices. They can be adjusted according to the individual needs and requirements and prove to be a helpful tool in veterinary practice health and safety management.

This chapter provides a clear framework for various topics of health and safety management in the veterinary practice.

18.1. INTRODUCTION

In recent years, general health and safety regulations as well as occupational health and safety policies and procedures have become an inevitable part of veterinary practice management. Apart from being a legal responsibility to create a safe workplace for the employees of the veterinary practice, occupational health and safety management should also be regarded as moral responsibility of all veterinary practitioners, veterinary practice owners and veterinary practice managers [18].

A special responsibility for veterinarians arises for non qualified veterinary staff, coworkers and lay staff as they are not sufficiently educated and informed about zoonotic diseases. It is therefore essential that veterinary practitioners take all adequate measures including awareness programs to ensure the health and safety of their staff. A failure to inform staff about potential diseases and their prevention may result in legal liabilities of the employers to the employee [8].

The introduction of health and safety procedures into daily practice life has an impact on preventing financial and legal liabilities and thus preventing possible high costs for the veterinary practice. In order to ensure the health and safety of staff, patients and patient owners, an overall safety program should be developed and implemented. It should be common in any practice to have an injury reporting systems as only then the frequency of individual incidents can be assessed and a prevention program can be established. An on-the-job interview is useful to perform the various duties successfully under consideration of health and safety policies and procedures.

18.2. ENVIRONMENTAL POLLUTION

Environmental pollution is an emerging issue in veterinary practices and hospitals. The nowadays existing codes of good veterinary practices intend to motivate veterinarians to reduce environmental pollution by waste avoidance [6]. This includes recycling and using re-usable articles when appropriate, and correct waste disposal. Another issue is disinfectants and cleaning chemicals that reach the water drainage.

Veterinarians should attempt to use disinfectants, medicinal products and other chemicals carefully and in the appropriate way. Economical use of energy and water is another help to avoid environmental pollution. Facilities for separate collection of different types of waste can be set up in order to send them to the appropriate recycling points. Disposal of infectious and non-infectious veterinary waste helps to reduce environmental pollutions [6]. However, environmental pollution happens not only in the waste and water sector but also in the air. In veterinary practices a major contributor to air pollution are anesthetic gases. They do not only lead to air pollution but also are potentially harmful for veterinary personnel. Correct use of anesthetic equipments and regular maintenance helps to reduce air pollution.

18.3. OCCUPATIONAL HEALTH
(ACUTE & CHRONIC HEALTH EFFECTS)

18.3.1. Nonparasitic Zoonotic Diseases

Nonparasitic zoonotic diseases pose 10% of all occupational injuries and diseases. In Australia, a survey revealed that 4% of the Australian veterinary practitioners have been infected with a zoonotic disease [11]. The outcomes of zoonotic diseases range from mild infections to fatal injuries [18]. Most common nonparasitic zoonotic diseases include cat scratch disease (bartonellosis), cat bite abscesses, Campylobacteriosis and dermatophytosis like ringworm.

Cat Scratches and Bites
Scratches and bites especially by cats should always be regarded as potentially infectious. They are normally more infectious than dog bites. Nevertheless, it is not possible to avoid cat or dog scratches or bites in a small animal practice. This shows a recent study stating that 3% to 18% of dog and 28% to 80% of cat bite wounds in humans have become infected [15].

However, through proper training of veterinary staff and application of correct handling and restraint techniques, the risk of such wounds can be greatly minimized. Personal protective measures like special gloves or restraint cages are also useful in case of already known aggressive and biting cats. As general rules, all scratches and bites should be cleaned and disinfected immediately. Immediate treatment is recommended for puncture wounds as they rank as high risk wounds. This applies especially wounds in the face, head, and hands as well as wounds with suspected involvement of tendons, nerves, or vascular structures [15].

Cat Scratch Disease (Bartonellosis)

Although regarded as zoonotic disease, cat scratches are not as dangerous as cat bites. Caused by the infectious agent *Bartonella henselae* or *B. clarridgeiae that is transmitted mainly by young kittens or feral cats, bartonellosis is normally characterized by a mild and self-limiting disease progress in humans [10].* Signs of clinical infection in humans typically range from development of a papule at the site of inoculation to regional lymphadenopathy, mild fever, malaise, and generalized myalgia. The latter usually shows spontaneously over a period of weeks to months [4, 10, 16].

Cat Bite Abscesses

Cat bite abscesses are a very common feature for veterinary practitioners. The problem is usually not the bite itself but the resulting secondary infections in which *Pasteurella* spp. are involved in approximately 75% of the cases [15]. Apart from *Pasteurella* spp., various other pathogens can be found in cat bite abscesses [15]. Despite the usually disease symptoms, serious health problems such as meningitis, recurrent abscesses, endocarditis, septic arthritis, septic shock and even death can be a result of cat bites [13, 15].

Campylobacteriosis

In humans, campylobacteriosis caused by *Campylobacter jejuni* has been stated as one of the most common causes of gastroenteritis and is mainly transmitted by infected dogs [18]. Clinical symptoms in humans may range from abdominal discomfort, fever and diarrhea that can be sometimes hemorrhagic. Antibiotic therapy is useful in such cases despite the fact that spontaneous recoveries are described. Although having mostly a mild disease process, in rare cases a serious demyelinating disease called trigger Guillain-Barre syndrome may arise.

Prevention of this clinical low prevalent infection is the avoidance of fecal-oral transmission [18].

Dermatophytosis

Dermatophytosis or commonly called ringworm describes a fungal infection caused by either *Trichophyton spp.* or *Microsporum spp.* This infection can be found in different animal species and especially in stray cats and highly populated catteries. Direct contact with infected animals, even asymptomatic carriers, leads to cutaneous lesion in humans after the 1 and 3 week incubation period [18]. Ringworm infections have been stated as most common zoonotic disease among British veterinarians [5]. Personal protection equipments like gloves and gowns should be used when handling infected animals [18].

18.3.2. Parasitic Zoonotic Diseases

Health and safety concerns may also arise in case of parasitic zoonotic diseases that might put veterinary personnel at risk. Those diseases include toxoplasmosis, giardiasis, and sarcoptes mange.

Toxoplasmosis

Infections with the coccidian parasite *Toxoplasma gondii* is mainly found in cats. Although often manifest in subclinical form, stressed or immune-compromised cats can also suffer from major clinical problems. Following the rare shedding of *T. gondii* oocysts, a low zoonotic potential arises for veterinary staff. However, the main problem of toxoplasmosis lies in the possible transmission to pregnant women and hereby especially pregnant veterinary staff. The reason is that *T. gondii* can cause congenital disease with spontaneous abortion, premature birth, encephalitis and neurological problems following an infection in the first and second pregnancy trimester. In veterinary personnel, such infection can occur through oral contact with contaminated cat feces. Therefore preventive measures include avoiding direct contact of pregnant veterinary staff with cat feces and especially cat litter as well as proper personal hygienic measures [19].

Giardiasis

As common cause for diarrhea in dogs and cats, *Giardia* infections are often found in young animals. Symptoms can range from asymptomatic infections to acute and chronic diarrhea. Humans get infected through contact with *Giardia* cysts in feces material. Typical symptoms in humans are diarrhea that can range from mild to severe and chronic forms. Preventive measures include proper hand washing and correct disposal of infected feces [19].

Sarcoptes Mange

Another parasitic disease in dogs is sarcoptes mange caused by *Sarcoptes scabiei* var. *canis*. As zoonotic transmission humans can be infected through *Sarcoptes scabiei* var. *canis*leading to either a self-limiting disease [19] or a persistent infection [3].

18.4. OCCUPATIONAL SAFETY (HAZARDOUS EXPOSURES)

A well functioning veterinary practice or hospital should have correct labeling and storage of medicines, consumables and hazardous items. This includes the Material Safety Data Sheets (MSDS) for e.g. all medicines and chemicals. They will provide information not only about the content, but also correct storage, safety information and hazardousness. All containers that are used in the veterinary practice should be correctly labeled to avoid wrong dispensing. This includes name of item, date of filling it in the containers, expiry date and if required dosage and application mode.

A written program preferably either in the veterinary practice/hospital management software or in excel sheets must include all information for medicines, consumables and hazardous items including their expiry date. Expired items should never be used and must be disposed according to the correct clinical and hazardous waste procedures. Furthermore, another written program should include the correct handling, frequency of use, transport and storage of e.g. disinfectants and pesticides.

Cross infection control recommendations and policies are very useful for veterinary practices in order to avoid cross contamination.

Despite the fact that the occupational health and safety procedures seem to be a lot of work in the beginning until they are completely set up, they can prove extremely valuable for the veterinary practice and its personnel but also in cases of disputes with external parties. Occupational health and safety procedures should be regarded as internal and external protective procedures for the veterinary practice and hospital. Once they are up and running, they can be easily continued and will become a normal part of the veterinary practice routine work.

18.5. PERSONAL INJURIES

The most common personal injury in the veterinary practice is bite wounds. Personal protective equipment should be available in any veterinary practice and the staff has to be fully trained to use them correctly. Other personal injuries contain slips, falls and trips. These can be caused by wet floors that are not properly marked as well as uneven surfaces in the practice premises.

Cuts can arise through unprofessional and careless handling of scalpel blades, knives and other cutting instruments. Often underestimated by veterinary personnel are injuries though manual handling. This happens especially when lifting heavy animals like big dogs or during restraint of animals.

Such injuries can be avoided through the use of hydraulic or electric examination and surgery tables, correct restraint procedures and sharing heavy weights with colleagues like carrying a big dog together. The correct ergonomic posture and movement also helps staff to avoid damage especially in their back region. It is well worth to train the veterinary staff in correct ways of handling, carrying and restraining animals as this will keep them healthier for a longer time.

Personal injuries in case of fire can be avoided by fire safety training as well as correct dealing with combustible substances. All possible fire and electric hazards have to be prevented in all areas of the veterinary practice or hospital. It is imperative that veterinary staff has to be made aware of possible fire and electrical hazards and their avoidance.

18.6. FATALITIES

Fatalities may be caused by nonparasitic zoonotic diseases like rabies. Other zoonotic infections contain leptospirosis, methicillin-resistant strains of *Staphylococcus aureus* (MRSA) and infections with Salmonella enterica sps enterica. However, fatalities may also arise through injuries and accidents.

18.6.1. Nonparasitic Zoonotic Diseases

Rabies

Rabies, a neurological disease caused by the Lyssa virus, poses a serious health threat for veterinary practitioners and their employees due to its high mortality rate. Worldwide more than 55,000 human deaths caused by rabies have been reported with dog bites amounting for 99% of those death cases [20]. Furthermore, rabies is re-emerging as a serious public health issue following recent human death increases caused by rabies in parts of Africa, Asia and Latin America [20].

The incubation period ranges from the typical 1–3 months to even up and more than 1 year. Rabies symptoms are fever, pain or an unusual or unexplained tingling as well as pricking or burning sensation (paraesthesia) at the wound site. The spreading of the Lyssa virus through the central nervous system results in progressive, fatal inflammation of the brain and spinal cord. The CNS infections results in two disease forms. The first one of furious rabies shows symptoms including hyperactivity, excited behavior, hydrophobia and sometimes aerophobia. Cardio-respiratory arrest leads to death after a few days [20]. The second form is the paralytic rabies that accounts for about 30% of the total number of human cases. This form is less dramatic and has usually longer course than the furious form. Signs are gradually paralyzed muscles that are starting at the site of the bite or scratch. A coma slowly develops, and eventually death occurs. The paralytic form of rabies is often misdiagnosed which leans to the underreporting of the disease [20].

Transmission occurs through bites or scratches of an infected animal being mainly dogs but also bats, when infectious material like saliva comes into contact with human mucosa or fresh skin wounds. Human rabies infections with subsequent deaths caused by foxes, raccoons, skunks, jackals, mongooses and other wild carnivores can be considered as very rare [20].

The best prevention of veterinary personnel is an updated rabies vaccination. Furthermore, wounds should be immediately cleaned and disinfected as well as undergo wound treatment following any bite or scratch.

Cat Bite Abscesses

As mentioned above in this chapter, cat bite abscesses may cause fatalities in humans [13, 15].

Leptospirosis

As one of the most widely distributed zoonotic diseases, leptospirosis is caused by the bacteria *Leptospira interrogans*. In animals, a peracute, acute and chronic form can be determined that in the worst case leads to death [7].

In humans, an infection can arise especially for veterinary staff through contact by urine. Another way of infection is the contamination though tissue of an infected animal with mucous membranes or skin lesions [16]. The disease can have a very varied clinical picture ranging from asymptomatic infections to death. Clinical symptoms in human beings include headache, nausea, myalgia and vomiting. Furthermore, more advanced symptoms can get manifest in the neurologic, cardiac, ocular and gastrointestinal systems [14, 12].

Leptospira infections in humans can be prevented by the use of gloves and barrier gowns when handing infected animals or items. Appropriate disinfection measures have to be taken in order to avoid animals or human contamination.

Salmonellosis

Salmonellosis caused by *Salmonella enterica sps enterica* results in systemic or enteric disease. Although dogs and cats can get infected from salmonellosis, they are not the major cause for Salmonella infections in humans. 90% and more of reptiles are carrying *Salmonella spp.* [17]. The strain *Salmonella* Typhimurium DT104 is of main concern to veterinary staff as it is a highly drug resistant strain [18] which has led to outbreaks in small animal practices. The main reasons for those outbreaks laid in problems with clinical and hygienic practices [1]. The fatal incidence in a human baby has been reportedly caused by a *Salmonella poona* infection in a pet reptile [2]. For this reason, veterinary personnel should be very cautious of a possible transmission of *Salmonella spp.* from animal patients to their children [18].

Disease prevention can be achieved through proper personal hygiene and hand washing techniques, identification of possible asymptomatic carriers among pets, surface disinfection and use of gloves when handling fecal material [18].

Methicillin-Resistant Staphylococcus Aureus

Methicillin-resistant *Staphylococcus aureus* (MRSA) strains have emerged as one of the major nosocomial infections not only in human hospitals, but also veterinary practices [18]. Although the percentage of infected veterinary personnel ranges from 9.7% to 17.9%, the infection has shown low incidence in non veterinary households. A higher incidence of MRSA positive veterinary staff has been reported in large animal practices [9]. Disease symptoms in humans include skin and soft tissue infections.

Prevention of MRSA can be achieved through careful personal hygiene like correct hand washing techniques, and alcohol based hand sanitizers.

18.6.2. Other Fatalities

Other work-related incidents that may lead to fatal results in veterinary personnel are mainly caused by accidents with animals. Veterinarians have died e.g. because of being kicked by a horse leading to a spleen rupture. The best prevention is careful handling of all animals and use of proper professional restraint procedures.

18.7. PROPERTY DAMAGES

Property damages may be caused by fire which can lead to major loss of buildings, equipments and profit. Fires might arise e.g. from defect machines, printers or equipments. Therefore all machinery and equipments in the veterinary practice should be routinely maintained to rule out such dangers. Correct fire-fighting equipment has to be in place and veterinary personnel have to be trained in fire drills how to react in case of fire and how to use fire-fighting equipments. Substantial claims might affect the practice if personal damage happens during a fire.

18.8. FINANCIAL AND LEGAL LIABILITIES

Financial liabilities may arise for the veterinary practice in cases where the occupational health and safety procedures have not been implemented and cause injuries or even fatalities either to staff, patients or customers. In order to protect the practice, well-designed occupational health and safety procedures are inevitable. Moreover, a good insurance should be covering all potential risks as the claims in case of injuries or fatalities might be much higher than the insurance rates!

18.9. CHECKLIST FOR OCCUPATIONAL HEALTH AND SAFETY MANAGEMENT IN THE VETERINARY PRACTICE/HOSPITAL

The following checklist for health and safety issues gives an example of how a workplace checklist can be set up for the individual veterinary practice. It should not be regarded as conclusive as each practice has special issues that should be included. In contrast, it is intended to provide ideas to the veterinary practice owner or practice manager to establish their own checklist for occupational health and safety management.

Table 18.1. Workplace checklist for occupational health and safety management in the veterinary practice/hospital

Issue	Yes	No	Remarks/Comments
1. Veterinary premises			
Is the practice/hospital maintained in safe, serviceable and hygienic condition?			
Does the practice/hospital have wheelchair ramps and proper access for disabled people?			
Are the adjacent kennels/stables connected to the main practice/hospital building?			
Do special intensive care units/isolation areas/quarantine exist?			
Are staff offices, food and recreation areas located away from treatment rooms, ICUs etc.?			
Are laboratory facilities located away from veterinary medical and staff areas?			
Is entry restricted to authorized staff only in all high risk areas like surgery/ ICUs/ quarantine/ laboratory/radiology?			
Are all computer cables etc. tied properly and removed from walking areas?			
Is the floor material not slippery?			
2. Veterinary Services			
Are veterinary services provided to dogs and cats?			
Are veterinary services provided to birds?			

Issue	Yes	No	Remarks/Comments
Are veterinary services provided to reptiles?			
Are veterinary services provided to horses?			
Are veterinary services provided to aggressive animals?			
Are veterinary services provided to stray animals?			
Are veterinary services provided to quarantined animals?			
Are high risk veterinary procedures conducted?			
Are necropsies conducted?			
3. Veterinary Staff			
Is staff vaccinated against tetanus?			
Do staff routinely disinfect cuts, bites or abrasions?			
Do staff routinely cover cuts, bites or abrasions?			
Do staff routinely wear disposable gloves when coming into contact with blood, wounds, feces, urine, mucous membranes etc.?			
4. Personnel protection equipment PPE			
Does the practice/hospital have PPEs for each staff as well as disposable PPEs?			
Does PPE include face masks, safety eyewear/shields, disposable gloves, disposable clothing, disposable footwear?			
Is protective clothing routinely worn when coming into contact with potentially infectious materials like droplets, blood, body substances?			
Is facial protection routinely worn when coming into contact with potentially infectious materials like droplets, blood, body substances?			
Are first aid kits available in each room of the veterinary practice/hospital?			
Are the first aid kits regularly checked and refilled if required?			
5. Training for health and safety			
Has veterinary and other personnel been trained routinely on health and safety procedures?			
Are training records kept?			
Is training mandatory for all staff?			
Are staff provided with health and safety information?			
Does new staff get health and safety induction?			
Are regular health and safety drills including fire alarm performed?			
6. Policies and Procedures			
Are occupational health and safety procedures in place?			
Are occupational health and safety procedures routinely revised and updated?			
Does a procedure for safe handling, storage, transport and disposal of clinical waste exist?			
Does a procedure for safe handling, storage, transport and disposal of clinical laundry exist?			
Does a hygiene procedure for cleaning and disinfection of rooms, premises and kennels/cages/stables exist?			
Does a hygiene procedure for cleaning and disinfection of veterinary instruments and equipments exist?			
Does a hygiene procedure for cleaning and disinfection of contaminated veterinary instruments and equipments exist?			

Table 18.1. (Continued)

Does ready access to hand hygiene amenities exist in all rooms of the practice/hospital including kennels/ stables?			
Does a procedure for sharp items exist?			
7. Hygiene and hygienic amenities			
Does personnel follow the hygiene procedures?			
Are hand hygiene amenities provided in the practice vehicles?			
Are foot baths available in high risk areas like quarantine?			
Are waste bins for infectious material clearly visible marked and with closed lids?			
Are areas where infectious animals have been examined/treated disinfected properly?			

18.10. CONCLUSION

Health and safety issues in the veterinary practice are a wide ranging and ever important topic. This includes environmental pollution especially with regard to clinical waste disposal as well as air pollution caused by anesthetic gases. Due to the special nature to the work, veterinary employees are subject to very serious occupational health risks like zoonotic diseases. These can be either caused by nonparasitic or parasitic zoonotic diseases that can range from clinical symptoms in affected humans. In the worst cases, zoonotic diseases may end up fatal.

The same applies to injuries as the work with animals results frequently in bites or other accidents. Those injuries can cause considerable damage to veterinary staff and can even lead to death. Occupational safety takes an increasing importance in the veterinary practice life. This includes correct labeling and storage of medicines, consumables and hazardous items as well as the use of Material Safety Data Sheets.

It is a good idea to establish a checklist for occupational health and safety management to understand and evaluate the various health and safety issues for veterinary premises, services, staff and hygiene. This aids in the trainings needs and setting up of policies and procedures. All those points lead to a responsible, reliable and accountable health and safety system that protects both, humans and animals.

REFERENCES

[1]   Anonymous (2001). Outbreaks of multidrug-resistant Salmonella typhimurium associated with veterinary facilities – Idaho, Minnesota, and Washington, 1999. *Morb. Mort. Wkly Rep.* 50 (33); pp. 701-704.

[2]   Anonymous (2000). Baby dies of Salmonella poona infection linked to pet reptile. *Commin. Dis. Rep. CDR Wkly*; 10. p. 161.

[3]   Arlian, L.G., Runyan, R.A. and Estes. S.A. (1984). Cross infectivity of sarcoptes scabiei. *J. Am. Acad. Dermatol.* 10; pp. 979-986.

[4] Breitschwerdt, E.B. and Greene, C.E. (1998). Bartonellosis. In: Greene CE, ed. *Infectious Diseases of the Dog and Cat*. 2nd ed. Philadelphia: WB Saunders. pp. 337–343.

[5] Constable, P.J. and Harrington, J.M. (1982). Risks of zoonoses in a veterinary service. *BMJ;* 284. pp. 246-248.

[6] FVE (2002). Federation of veterinarians in Europe. Code of good veterinary practice. http://www.fve.org/news/publications/pdf/gvp.pdf(Accessed on August, 14th, 2011).

[7] Greene, C.E., Miller, M.A. and Browne, C.A. (1998). Leptospirosis. In: Greene, C.E. ed. Infectious diseases of the dog and cat. 2nd. Ed. Philadelphia: WB. Saunders. pp. 273-281.

[8] Hannah, H.W. (1994). A veterinarian's liability to employees. *J. Am. Vet. Med. Assoc.* 204. pp. 361–362.

[9] Hanselman, B.A., Kruth, S.A., Rousseau, J., Low, D.E., Willey, B.M., McGreer, A. and Weese, J.S. (2007). Methicillin-resistant Staphylococcus aureus colonization in veterinary personnel. *Emerg. Inf. Dis.* 12; pp. 1933-1938.

[10] Harrington, K.S. and Groves, M.S. (1995). Cat scratch disease. In: Farris R, Mahlow J, Newman E, Nix B, eds. Health Hazards in Veterinary Practice. 3rd ed. Austin, Texas: *Texas Department of Health.* pp. 23–24.

[11] Jeyaretnam, J., Jones, H., Phillips, M. (2000). Disease and injury among veterinarians. *Vet. J.* August (78). pp. 625–629.

[12] Levett, P.N. (2001). Leptospirosis. *Clin. Microbiol. Rev.,* 14; pp. 296-326.

[13] Love, D.N., Malik, R. and Norris, J.M. (2000). Bacteriologic warfare amongst cats: what have we learned about cat bite infections? *Vet. Microbiol.* 74. pp. 179–193.

[14] Roth, R.M. and Gleckman, R.A. (1985). Human infections derived from dogs. *Postgrad. Med.* 77; pp. 169-180.

[15] Talan, D.A., Citron, D.M., Abrahamian, F.M., Moran, G.J. and Goldstein, E.J.C. (1999). Bacteriologic analysis of infected dog and cat bites. *N. Engl. J. Med.* 340. pp. 85–92.

[16] Tan, J.S. (1997). Human zoonotic infections transmitted by dogs and cats. *Arch. Intern. Med.* 157. pp. 1933–1943.

[17] Ward, L. (2000). Salmonella perils of pet reptiles. *Comm. Dis. Pub. Health.* 31. pp. 2-3.

[18] Weese, J.S., Peregrine, A.S. and Armstrong, J. (2002a). Occupational health and safety in veterinary practices. Part I -Nonparasitic zoonotic diseases. *Can. Vet. J.* August (43)8. pp. 631-636.

[19] Weese, J.S., Peregrine, A.S. and Armstrong, J. (2002b). Occupational health and safety in veterinary practices. Part II -Parasitic zoonotic diseases. *Can. Vet. J.* August (43)8. pp. 799-802.

[20] WHO (2010). (World Health Organization) Rabies. Fact sheet N°99. Updated September 2010. http://www.who.int/mediacentre/factsheets/fs099/en/ (Accessed on June 18th, 2011).

Chapter 19

RISK ANALYSIS AND EMERGENCY PREPAREDNESS

ABSTRACT

A risk analysis considers internal and external risk factors and is essential to be carried out before setting up the business. It helps to control negative impacts on the business that can affect the veterinary practice either from inside or outside. Some factors cannot be influenced like legal and economic changes, but a risk analysis can visualize the impact and assess the effects on business. One frequently used risk analysis is the SWOT analysis that provides an overview of the strengths, weaknesses, opportunities and threats of businesses. It is applicable to veterinary practices and hospitals, too. The same applies to risk assessment plan as well as emergency preparedness plans. This chapter provides a clear framework for risk analysis, risk assessment and emergency preparedness management in the veterinary practice.

19.1. INTRODUCTION

"Risk management is the process of conserving earning power and assets by minimizing the shock from losses" [3]. There are two types of risk being voluntarily undertaken risks and unavoidable risks. The risks being voluntarily undertaken are uncertainties, the so-called speculative risks. Nevertheless, there are certain strategies to cope with the risk or to reduce it. One choice is to refuse to take a risk which might be too costly thus avoiding the risk [3]. This might be applicable to the introduction of new and expensive services or purchase of expensive equipment when it is not sure if a sufficient customer clientele is available [4].

Another strategy is to control the losses by prevention through e.g. work safety measures [3]. Insurances serve as risk transfer when the risk is transferred from the business to an outside entity, e.g. the insurer company [3].

A very useful strategy is the self-insurance where the business might set a certain amount of money aside to meet unexpected and uncertain losses [3]. This can cover smaller damages in the practice or small practice car damages, which need to be replaced immediately and are not too costly [4].

19.2. INTERNAL RISK FACTORS FOR THE VETERINARY PRACTICE

The internal risk factors of the practice can be evaluated with a so-called SWOT analysis identifying the strengths, weaknesses, opportunities and threats. Important areas for a SWOT analysis in the veterinary practice are premises, location, services, products, clients, marketing, finance, competitor situation, legislation, managements systems and IT support [6].

The strengths of a business are its brand name, an excellent distribution network as well as skilled and loyal employees. Weaknesses can be the lack of new products, the high amount of costs and borrowing. However, good opportunities for a business might be new market openings due to political or economic change as well as development of new technologies. Nevertheless, the business can be threatened by economic or legislative changes as well as new strong competitors. This analysis will be ideally conducted in all areas of the business [3, 4].

Table 19.1. SWOT analysis for veterinary practice [4]

Strengths	Opportunities
1. Brand name 2. Wide range of services 3. Specialist services 4. Dedicated employees with expertise 5. Good and central location 6. Loyal clientele 7. Highly populated catchment area	1. New markets due to economic change 2. New technology 3. Additional market shares through new innovative services 4. Good premises with space for expansion 5. New clients through new services
Weaknesses	Threats
1. Lack of new services 2. High costs 3. High level of borrowing 4. Lack of marketing 5. Lack of professional IT structure 6. Lack of business planning skills	1. Economic change/recession 2. New competitors 3. Change in legislation 4. Change in partnership/owner structure 5. Reduction of farm animals 6. Internet veterinarians and veterinary product sales

19.3. EXTERNAL RISK FACTORS FOR THE VETERINARY PRACTICE

External risk factors cannot be influenced and are divided into political, environmental, social and technological factors [5]. The political and legal environment might have influence on environmental and health and safety laws as well as prices and taxes. Those political and legal factors might be changes in legislation or qualification requirements [5], which can affect the veterinary practice when e.g. changes in the veterinary qualifications occur. Health and safety standards [1] might also have a special influence on the daily veterinary work.

In contrast, the social environment includes the demographic situation, lifestyles, social values and cultural factors. The other external risk factor, the economic environment will be influenced by economic growth rates, productivity, inflation and interest rates. Technological risk and threats can derive from new emerging technologies, technological capabilities and research and development. The physical or environmental risks cover pollution, global weather trends and warming and energy prices [1].

A risk strategy is to control the losses by prevention through e.g. work safety measures [3] which is especially consequential in the veterinary practice where health and safety measures are extremely important due to the infectious environment and zoonotic diseases. In the practice, e.g. carelessness with contagious material might lead to sick leave of staff and possible employment of expensive locum staff. This leads not only to financial losses, but also to staff health damage and uncertainty among the remaining staff about the safety of their workplace. Insurances serving as risk transfer [3] are a highly important feature in the veterinary practice life as veterinarians and veterinary employees have an extremely high risk of professional disability incurred during work. This can lead to permanent disability making it impossible for the veterinarian or veterinary staff to work in a practice again or even to work at all. These risks need to be covered in order not to fall through the social network completely. Risk transfers to insurances might help also in-law cases due to alleged malpractice, which can go into large amounts of money if a valuable animal was affected.

Environmental or physical factors might be a natural disaster like storms, pollution or flooding. The latter might affect the veterinary practice directly, not only by the water which might destroy the practice interior but also by a large number of dead animals and therefore, loss of clientele.

Social threats for the veterinary practice are posed by a decreasing pet population thus leading to a reduced clientele. Other social threats for veterinarians are the demographic situation with fewer children in the families. Usually especially children prefer to have a pet and many families keep pets only for them. A further imbalance of younger and very old people will have an influence on the development of veterinary practices in the future.

Economic factors like a recession period might severely affect the veterinary practice as people will not spend as much money as before on their pet's health as they simply cannot afford it anymore. Other economical factors are the influence of major animal diseases like foot-and-mouth disease or Avian Influenza which has led to tremendous losses in the livestock and poultry sector in recent years. This has not only affected the farmers but also the veterinary practices alike.

19.4. RISK ASSESSMENT

A risk assessment should be performed in every veterinary practice. It identifies potential risks in the workplace like accidents, damages as well as hazards that can cause harm to employees and other people. However, what is a hazard and what is a risk? A hazard is everything that might result in harm like electricity, chemicals, falling over cables, bites or slipping. The risk is the chance, no matter how high or low, that a person or animal can be harmed by such hazards as well as any other hazards. It indicates the seriousness of the harm.

The risk assessment covers risk potentials for veterinary personnel as well as patients and clients. Avoidable accidents can cause permanent disabilities and even death. Furthermore, accidents, injuries or machine and equipment damage might cause considerable costs for the veterinary practice with future increased insurance rates. In the worst case, they might even lead to judicial consequences like court cases. Moreover, from a legal point of view, veterinary practices are required to have risk assessments to protect their staff and facilities. Therefore, the risk assessment has to be performed before designing the emergency preparedness plan.

In the health sector, risk assessments are often including hazard assessments or hazard vulnerability analysis.

Risks can be classified as e.g.:

- Threat to life or health
- Disruption of services
- Damage or failure possibilities
- Financial impact
- Legal issues
- Loss of community trust

How can risk be assessed in a step-by-step approach? When making the risk assessment, it is always better to keep it simple and easily understandable as all employees have to understand and be trained on it.

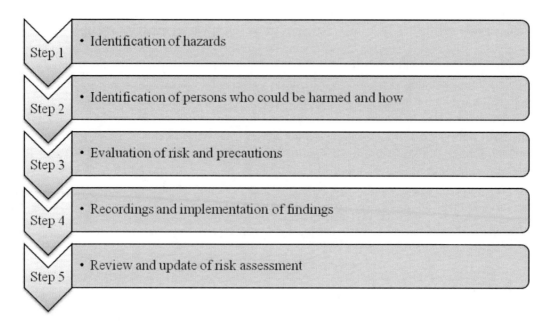

- Step 1 • Identification of hazards
- Step 2 • Identification of persons who could be harmed and how
- Step 3 • Evaluation of risk and precautions
- Step 4 • Recordings and implementation of findings
- Step 5 • Review and update of risk assessment

Figure 19.1. Step-by-step risk assessment [modified from 2].

In step 1, the practice owner or manager should go around the veterinary practice to see if he can identify hazards such as hanging computer cables, open chemicals or damaged cages. It is always good to seek the input of employees as they might have recognized potential risk areas that might not be very evident [2]. Long-term hazards to health like exposure to X-ray beams or anesthesia gases should not be left out. Moreover, records of previous accidents and injuries can be included [2]. In most countries, official health and safety websites do exist for veterinary use.

Step 2 identifies persons who could be harmed by each hazard, which can vary among different hazards [2]. Apart from veterinary practice personnel, clients, cleaners, maintenance people, contractors, suppliers, etc. have to be taken into consideration. Animals should not be left out as we are talking here of a risk assessment for the veterinary practice!

In the third step, the veterinary practice owner or manager needs to decide how to evaluate the hazards and risk and what precautions can be taken to prevent them. First of all, it needs to be decided whether the hazards can be completely eradicated or if not, how it can be contained [2]. This includes the implementation for a less risky option such as changing one acid chemical against a less acid one [2].

Personal protection equipment can be used very well to reduce potential risks through hazards [2]. Warning sign, e.g. wet floor or biting dog can help to prevent damages. Restricted access to hazard areas, e.g. laboratory or barriers in- between, e.g. security doors can greatly reduce risk. Sometimes such precautions might be fairly cheap but can be used to a great effect.

Moreover, veterinary staff should be integrated in the process as they might come up with very practical and creative idea as they see the work place from an entirely perspective as the practice owner or manager.

Step 4 is the time when all findings will be written up in the risk assessment sheet [2]. This exercise is best done together with the staff. It is useful to keep the write up simple and precise.

The risk plan should include quick wins like smaller things that can be implemented easily with low costs and larger changes that require planning at a higher cost. It is important to let actions follow the establishing of the risk assessment plan. Otherwise the whole exercise is simply for nothing, and the practice owner or manager will lose credibility among staff. The last step is the readjustment of the plan to a new situation [2] like moving to new premises or purchase of latest equipments. A review should be performed on an annual basis.

The information gathered in the risk assessment plan will flow into the emergency preparedness plan.

19.5. EMERGENCY PREPAREDNESS PLAN

Every veterinary practice should have an emergency preparedness plan, at least a basic one. It helps to react in crisis situations like natural disaster or other emergencies in a controlled way.

An emergency preparedness plan includes several components:

- Emergency Preparedness Plan
- Communication
- Distribution of staff responsibilities
- Training

- Drills
- Evacuation plan
- Internal disaster procedures, e.g. for fire
- Annual evaluation

Every emergency preparedness plan contains three categories, probability, risk and preparedness. Other categories or events can be added if required. Issues that need to be considered in the various categories include the following:

Table 19.2. Issues to be considered for probability, risk and preparedness

Probability	Risk	Preparedness
Known risk	Threat to life or health	Status of current plans
Historical data	Disruption of services	Training status
Manufacturer statistics	Damage or failure possibilities	Availability of backup systems
Vendor statistics	Financial impact	Insurance
	Legal issues	Resources
	Loss of community trust	

The emergency preparedness plan includes various scores for the likelihood of events and their grades. For all emergencies, emergency electricity e.g. generator and water supplies should be available.

Table 19.3. Sample emergency preparedness plan

Event	Probability				Risk					Preparedness			Total
	High	Med	Low	None	Life threat	Health safety	High disruption	Moderate Disruption	Low disruption	Poor	Fair	Good	
Score	3	2	1	0	5	4	3	2	1	3	2	1	
Natural events													
Severe thunderstorm													
Snow													
Ice													
Blizzard													
Tornado													
Hurricane													
Flood													
Drought													
Wildfire													
Landslide													
Technological events													

Event	Probability				Risk					Preparedness			Total
	High	Med	Low	None	Life threat	Health safety	High disruption	Moderate Disruption	Low disruption	Poor	Fair	Good	
Score	3	2	1	0	5	4	3	2	1	3	2	1	
Electrical failure													
Generator failure													
Water failure													
Heating failure													
Fire alarm failure													
Transportation failure													
Communications failure													
Information system failure													
Oxygen failure													
Fire internal													
Flood internal													
Hazmat exposure internal													
Supply failure													
Structural damage													
Human events													
Injuries													
Accidents													
Demographic changes													
Sabotage													
Civil disorder													
Pandemics													
Threatening behavior													
Violent behavior													
Criminal behavior													

The evacuation plan needs to be set up. This includes the delegation of authorities in case of an emergency, e.g. practice owner or manager will give the order to evacuate the practice facilities. The evacuation should include all humans and if possible time wise, animal patients.

All veterinary personnel have to be trained on that plan, and drills have to be conducted routinely, preferable every six months. The emergency preparedness training will include specific roles and responsibilities during emergencies and communication. Skills that are required to perform duties during emergencies have to be especially trained.

19.6. CONCLUSION

The veterinary practice can be affected by internal as well as external risks. Internal risks can be partly avoided through proper planning and correct forecasting as well as controlling the market fluctuations. They can be evaluated with the SWOT analysis that identifies the strengths, weaknesses, opportunities and threats of the veterinary business. This is even more important is a fast-paced changing business world with increasing competitors. Such a SWOT analysis should be undertaken for all areas of business as this can lead to different results requiring distinctive actions.

External factors might pose a risk for the veterinary practice but cannot be avoided. Therefore, measures to contain them have to be put in place. This requires, firstly, a risk assessment and secondly, a plan to tackle those risks. Although risk assessment sounds very complicate, it is not if a step-by-step approach is taken. It is something that can be undertaken in every veterinary practice as a team exercise.

Once the first risk assessment has been performed it only needs to be revised on annual basis. The benefits of the risk assessment outweigh the time invested in developing it for the first time. And we should not forget that it is in the veterinary practice owner's responsibility to provide a safe and as much as possible risk-free work environment for staff. The risk assessment flows into the emergency preparedness plan which helps to react in correct way in case of emergencies, no matter of which kind. Risk assessment and emergency preparedness plans round up the health and safety management of veterinary practices.

REFERENCES

[1]   Cairns, G., Moore, C., Reid, C. Scouller, J. and Wilkie, R. (2006). *Exploring the business environment. Rev. ed.* The Graduate School of Business, University of Strathclyde, Glasgow, UK.

[2]   HSE (2011). Health and Safety Executive. Five steps to risk assessment.http://www.hse.gov.uk/pubns/indg163.pdf (Accessed on August, 18th, 2011).

[3]   Megginson, W.L., Byrd, M.J. and Megginson, L.C. (2000). Small business management: *An entrepreneur's guidebook.* 3rd ed. McGraw-Hill. Boston, Madrid, Toronto.

[4]   Müller, M.G. and Abu Aabed, A. (2007). Guidelines for setting up a small and medium size enterprise. *MBA Thesis, University of Strathclyde.* Graduate School of Business. Glasgow, UK.

[5]   Reuvid, J. and Millar, R. (2003). Start up & run your own business. 2nd ed. *Abbey National Business.* Kogan Page.London. UK.

[6]   Shilcock, M. and Stutchfield, G.(2008). Veterinary practice management. *A practical guide.* 2nd ed. Saunders, Elsevier Ltd. Philadelphia.

Chapter 20

SUCCESSFUL GROWTH OF THE VETERINARY PRACTICE

ABSTRACT

The successful growth of the veterinary practice is vital for the survival and profitability of veterinary practices in a fast-paced changing world. This chapter provides a structured approach of identifying the growth potential of a practice in an easily applicable systematic approach. The way of introducing successfully new services as well as possible pitfalls are explained in detail. Proper planning of new services and market analysis is crucial. Apart from existing core business areas of veterinary practices, new business pillars should be added to enhance the survival rate and to increase growth and profitability even in economic difficult times. This modern vision of modular veterinary practice models is detailed with examples in this chapter.

20.1. INTRODUCTION

It can be a challenging task to maneuver the veterinary practice successfully through good times and especially through difficult economic times. Challenges can be growing revenues and profit, increased client satisfaction and increased market competition. However, the survival of veterinary practices depends on their abilities to improve their market position even when times are rough. But how can this survival be achieved?

When looking at growth of successful companies with regard to revenue and value acquisition, a differentiation in four categories can be found: growth giants, performers, unrewarded and challenged [2].

Growth giants are those businesses that have outperformed in both, revenue and value. Performers have increased value but did not improve revenues whereas the unrewarded businesses have outperformed in revenue but not in value. Challenged are described as those companies with lack in both, revenue and value [2].

In subsequent business cycles, growth giants persevered and extended their growth whereas performers declined. On the other hand, challenged companies perked up and unrewarded ones sustained uncertainty [2]. Although the "grow or go" dynamics has been established mainly for large companies, it can be applied to veterinary practices as small business entities. In which part of the matrix would you like your veterinary practice to be? Growth giants? This requires hard and clever work but it is possible to achieve it.

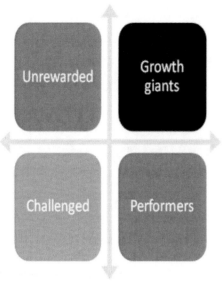

Figure 20.1. The growth performance matrix [modified from 2].

20.2. IDENTIFYING AREAS OF GROWTH POTENTIAL

How do we look at veterinary business markets? Do we regard them as one whole market or as segmented markets? The so-called granularity model regards individual small components in the bigger market picture [2] and can help veterinary practices to build areas of strength and subsequent growth.

The granularity model identifies different areas of growth potential in businesses. They include:

- Expansion of customer segment by seeking to attract other customer markets [2]
- Expansion in product segment by targeting other buying needs of customers [2]
- Expansion in a wider geographic area by entering in new markets [2]

This can be adopted very well for the veterinary business structure. Veterinary practices can seek for growth through:

- Expansion of client segments by seeking to attract other clients markets, e.g. opening of avian services if there are several bird breeders in the catchment area
- Expansion in product segments by targeting other client needs and consumer behavior, e.g. opening of pet grooming and boarding services
- Expansion in a wider geographic area by identifying new service segments in new markets, e.g. opening of specialist referral services

Before embarking on a growth strategy, the veterinary practice owner needs to decide whether the practice wants to go for a short-term win or long-term sustainable growth. Market shares have more influence over shorter periods like one-year periods but do not contribute to the long-term growth performance of companies [2]. A long-term strategy for the growth of the veterinary practice is a more viable approach. The so-called horizon model [2] can be modified for veterinary practices:

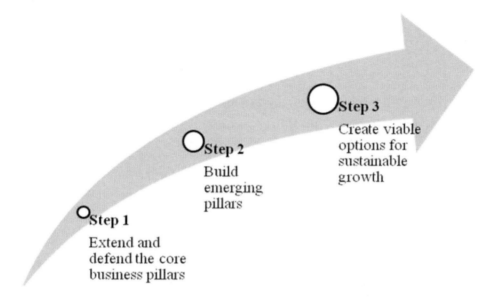

Figure 20.2. Growth of veterinary business [modified from 2].

In step 1, the core strength of the veterinary business is subject to expansion. It needs to be protected and defended against a possible decline as most of the profit and cash flow derives from this business segment [2]. The core business pillars provide necessary resources for growth [2] and short-term as well as long-term performance. In order to grow this business part, available resources should be allocated to the department or unit with the highest growth potential. This includes money for required investments, leadership talents and faster decision-making authorities [2].

The second step of building emerging business pillars describes the development of service and business lines that are still in the future and will pay off in the end [2]. Far-sighted veterinary practice owners should keep these provisions in mind, as it is not sufficient for sustainable growth just to focus on the existing business segments. They have to be creative, innovative and visionary as these are the essential traits for business expansion and subsequent business success.

The third step, the creation of viable options for future progression are small areas that might not yet be matching the practice portfolio or that require testing phases or start as smaller project. However, they can become alternatives with high potential in future [2]. It is sufficient in the beginning to start those services on a small scale and then develop them in the way that is more progressive after the initial successful testing phase. Moreover, veterinary practice owners and managers have to be open-minded in the modern business world to see and catch prospective new business ideas.

20.3. Introduction of New Services and Products

After having identified the areas of business growth, it is time to think of introducing new services. Before their setting up, it is important to understand the needs and requirements of the clients. It is always easier to introduce new services to existing clients as they know and appreciate the professionalism and quality of the veterinary practice. The second reason for new service introduction is the assumption that the clients' demand for the new service is high enough to make it profitable. There is no need to open a new business line when it does not increase revenues and profits. Moreover, the new service has to match the general portfolio of the practice, at least in the beginning until the side pillars are strong enough to support the core business. This means it is not helpful to introduce dog grooming in a pure equine practice, as it does not have the right clientele. However, as viable options for future progression new service and product options can be gathered even if they do not form part of the core and side pillars of the practice yet.

Before introducing a new business line or service, it is vital to study and estimate the potential market and to be aware of possible pitfalls. A wrong step in this directions leads inevitable to the failure of the business [1]. Another reason for the failure of new services or products is the fact that the same item was offered as the competitors just to follow them. Wrong estimates of the development of the new service or product above the planned budget lead to failure. Incorrectly positioned products that are not matching the market do not succeed due to lacking demand. The same applies to too expensive or poorly designed services that do not find acceptance by the clientele. Furthermore it can be crucial to underestimate competitors as they will fight back to protect their own business [1].

In contrast, well-designed new services can be introduced with great success. This requires excellent preparation before their introduction. First, a thorough market analysis with customer requirements identification has to be conducted followed by setting up of a strong concept [1]. The benefits of the new service have to be established. Introduction of new technology and meeting of clients' needs have to be matched [1]. In order to succeed with the introduction of a new service or product in the veterinary practice, the service or product has to be evaluated from all different angles including client views, financial feasibility, design, marketing and pricing.

Before embarking on a new service, the practice owner or manager has to evaluate if the practice has sufficient capacities. If this is not the case, the preparation for new services might include a professional specialization on a potentially viable service area like dentistry, ophthalmology or specific surgery methods. Furthermore, proficient training of employees on the new service is vital to make it a professional quality service. They need to understand its benefits to convince the clients. Once practice members see the potential advantage of the new service or product, they will be much more motivated to introduce it to the customers and their positive aura will translate to them.

In general, new services take about three to five years to grow and mature. By that time, they can become very profitable and develop to a strong and profitable pillar of the veterinary practice. If the practice owner or manager realizes a need to grow the business within the next 3-5 years, he should start already to pave the way for it. It should be taken into consideration that new services cannot be introduced to a successful level overnight.

The best way forward to introducing new services or products in the veterinary practice is to start it small and test it among the clients. The veterinary practice needs to train its clients in using the new services. Compliments and praise or rewards achieve this in the introduction phase. Once the clients are used to the new services and embrace them, profit will come by itself. Satisfied customers will make word-by-mouth marketing for the new services leading to an increased awareness of the new service even among a new potential customer clientele. Whenever the practice introduces a new service or product, clients need to understand the direct correlation of the new services and its positive influence on improved healthcare of their animals. This is the key success factor for new service and products that cannot be stressed enough. It is not just about the fact that the veterinary practice introduces the new services, it is more about how it offers and publicizes them. If this marketing part is conducted successfully, the new offerings can be expanded without the risk of losing too much money. This strategy can lead to good returns on investment with controlled risk.

20.4. MODULAR VETERINARY PRACTICE MODELS

The old and previously very successful veterinary practice model has to pay tribute to the ever-changing economic and demographic situations that have greatly affected the veterinary business world in recent years. Although it was a perfect model in previous years, it will not be strong enough to counter those major changes.

The veterinary practice model of the future is the modular veterinary practice that stands on several pillars. The modular veterinary practice can be composed of general veterinary services as main pillar and core business area with additional modules of different service offerings. Those side pillars can be differently developed and advanced. They can also bring different amount of revenues. It is only important that they help to support the veterinary business as a whole.

Even in economic difficult times, some pillars will grow and help to sustain or further grow the veterinary business with increased revenue and profit whereas other pillars will decline, possibly temporarily.

The establishing of a modular veterinary practice model does not mean that the veterinary surgeon has to perform all services by him alone. It rather indicates that nursing or receptionist staff can do several new services like grooming, pet nutrition advice or sale of pet accessories. This uses their abilities more than before which leads to increased staff motivation as well as profitability.

Even large veterinary hospitals or specialist referral hospitals can benefit from the modular veterinary practice model. If we take a surgery referral center as example, we can apply the model by adding new services that are related to surgery and complement it. Adding to the core business of general surgery, new pillars like neurology, ophthalmology, dentistry and oral surgery will provide a matching but wider service offering. Other possibilities of new services are in this context e.g. physiotherapy and acupuncture.

This model is applicable to all kind of veterinary practices and hospitals and can be amended easily to fit the current situation as well as qualifications of the veterinary practice team.

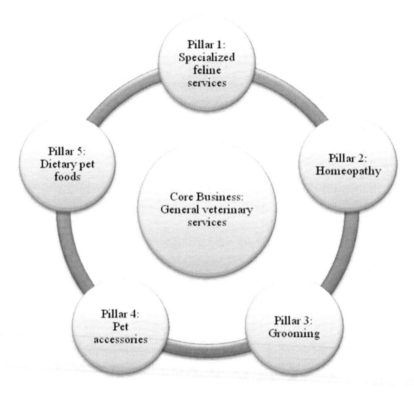

Figure 20.3. Modular small animal practice model.

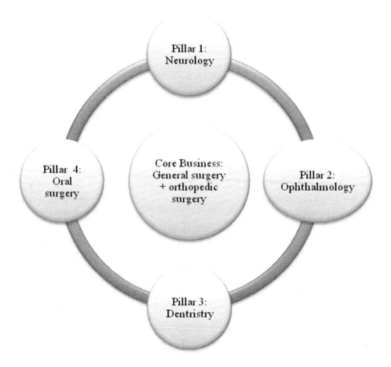

Figure 20.4. Modular veterinary referral surgery model.

20.5. Conclusion

Modern business life and fast-paced economic changes as well as demographic changes lead to an adaptation of veterinary practice models to those new circumstances. Growth in veterinary practices can only be achieved if the practice is standing on several pillars that support and complement each other. Before introducing new services, performing a market study helps to identify growth potential, even if this is possible only on a smaller scale. Well-planned services are introduced first on smaller scale to test the clients' reactions. Then they will be rolled out on larger scale. It usually takes 3-5 years to turn a new service into a profitable practice pillar with strong growth and future development perspectives. The newly introduced modular veterinary practice model helps in balancing various service offerings to achieve growth.

It helps to protect the practice from economic crisis, as always one of those pillars will be able to be more profitable while other decline. Nowadays veterinary practices have to be much more pro-active due to increased competition. Veterinarians need to seek actively for new opportunities. This includes the fact that they themselves have to review their own knowledge and skills and, if necessary, enhance them through professional education and special training courses.

This will benefit them and subsequently the veterinary practice. Life-long learning stands hand in hand with the growth of modern veterinary practices and provide the basis for the modular veterinary practice model. Veterinary practice owners and practitioners have to adhere to current changes in the veterinary business world if they want to succeed and grow their business in future. They need to adopt a business-oriented vision that supports them economically and enhances patients' care to highest levels in the same time. The modular veterinary practice model being presented in this chapter supports both sides in a comprehensive and future-oriented way.

References

[1]   Scott, J.T. (2009). The Entrepreneur's guide to building a successful business. *Management Education Services.*

[2]   Viguerie, P., Smit, S. and Baghai, M. (2010). Granularity. Smart choices to grow your business in good times and bad. *Marshall Cavendish Business.* London, UK.

Chapter 21

EXCELLENCE IN VETERINARY PRACTICE

ABSTRACT

Excellence is in the business world is a concept that is successfully implemented in many international companies. However, it does not yet play an important role in the veterinary business world. Veterinary practices can greatly benefit from introducing excellence in their daily work routine. This chapter details the road to excellence for veterinary practices in a systematic approach. The various steps to achieve excellence are explained in detail. Special emphasis is put on important improvement areas in the veterinary practice as this provides the framework for excellence. Furthermore, the role of employees in the change process is highlighted, as their acceptance is critical for the successful implementation of excellence. This chapter aims at motivating veterinary practice owners and managers to start the journey to excellence and outperform themselves to the benefit of their patients.

21.1. INTRODUCTION

The previous chapters of this book provided information about the setting up of a veterinary practice and described the main issues of veterinary practice management. Now we come to the overall important topic of how to survive in a market with ever-increasing competition. This raises the question of how the veterinary practice can be unique. This chapter will introduce the reader to the concept of excellence to create the veterinary practice as an outstanding business. What is excellence in general and more specifically in the veterinary business context?

Excellence has been defined as "The quality of being excellent; state of possessing good qualities in an eminent degree; exalted merit; superiority in virtue" and "An excellent or valuable quality; that by which any one excels or is eminent; a virtue" [2]. This definition is applicable not only to general businesses, but to veterinary practices alike. Astonishingly, veterinary practice routine and thinking have not yet integrated excellence very much in all its forms although they strive to improve patient care. As competition gets tougher and tougher, practices have to increase their competitive advantage to attract a wider customer clientele. How is this achievable? Veterinary practices that embrace excellence integrate it in all parts of their daily routine. It is not a onetime commitment; in contrast, excellence demands an ongoing desire to outperform in order to serve the patients and clients in the best possible way.

21.2. EXCELLENCE IN VETERINARY PRACTICE

The topic of excellence in veterinary practices is a very new one. Although being established since long time in the business world, excellence is just entering the veterinary world. As excellent service providers outperform themselves, veterinary practices and their clients can benefit greatly from upgrading their good service offerings to excellent service offerings. To reach out for excellence is an ongoing journey and demands the commitment of each team member.

In recent years, veterinary organizations have come up with the introduction of codes of good veterinary practice conduct to improve work ethics and to introduce quality management measures [1]. Covering general principles, those guidelines can be used as an aid in going for quality certifications like e.g. ISO certification [1]. However, those codes are not legally binding and depend on the voluntarily integration of those principles.

When looking at excellence in the veterinary practice, it becomes evident that the road to excellence is long and better be broken down in smaller steps. Therefore, the main steps to achieve excellence in the veterinary practice are outlined as follows:

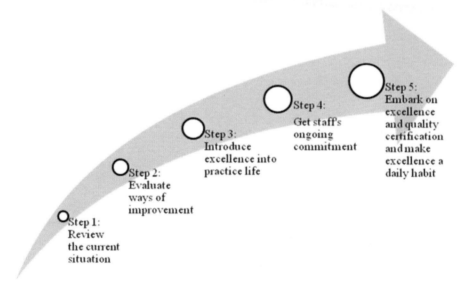

Figure 21.1. The way to excellence in veterinary practice.

21.2.1. Step 1 to Excellence

The first step on the way to excellence in veterinary practice is the review of the current situation. The progressive practice is pro-active to find out what clients need and how to respond positively to external changes. This can include a client survey and comments by customers. The revenue and income are examined for areas of bigger growth or decline over time. Core business parts are identified and evaluated. One great way to understand the current situation is simply asking the employees about their opinion. They have a different point of view and might come up with ideas of improvement that a practice owner or manager will not necessarily think of. Review of the current situation takes place in the four main areas of excellence:

❖ Customers
  • Patient care
  • Client satisfaction
  • Compliance and number of revisits
  • Range of services and products
  • Complaints
❖ Employees
  • Employees satisfaction and motivation
  • Employees workload
❖ Practice operations
  • Workflow and processes
  • Waiting time
  • Status of equipments and machinery
  • Introduction of new services
  • Income and profitability
  • Facilities and premises
❖ Leadership
  • Perception of senior staff
  • Perception of employees

21.2.2. Step 2 to Excellence

The second step is to evaluate areas and ways of improvement. Every veterinary practice has areas that require many efforts to improve the standards. Although it sounds boring and time consuming, it is worth checking out each area and to ask what could be improved to enhance patient care and client satisfaction and to speed up workflow.

❖ **Customers**
  • Can patient care be improved and how?
    ➢ Better equipments
    ➢ Better staff knowledge
    ➢ Better facilities
    ➢ New medicines
  • Can client satisfaction be improved and how?
    ➢ Review of client satisfaction survey and evaluation of trends

- ➤ Reduced waiting time
- ➤ Better treatment methods
- ➤ Clearer instructions and recommendations during consultations
- ➤ Better appointment scheduling e.g. e-bookings
- ➤ Wider range of services
- ➤ Opening of new service segments e.g. behavior advice, nutrition, in-house laboratory testing
- ➤ Introduction of pick-up service
- ➤ Introduction of home visits
- ➤ Comprehensive merchandising
- Compliance and number of revisits
  - ➤ How many clients are coming again?
  - ➤ How many revisits are required to cure the patient?
  - ➤ Do animal owners follow the veterinarian's instructions?
  - ➤ Do clients come for re-vaccination appointments?
- Range of services and products
  - ➤ Is the range of services and products sufficient?
  - ➤ Can existing services be improved and how?
- Complaints
  - ➤ How many complaints are received?
  - ➤ Who complains?
  - ➤ What is the reason for complaints?
  - ➤ Are complaints justified?
  - ➤ How can complaints be reduced?
  - ➤ Does management take complaints seriously?
  - ➤ Do employees take complaints seriously?
  - ➤ How is the reaction on complaints?
  - ➤ What can be changed to reduced complaints?

❖ **Employees**
- Employees satisfaction and motivation
  - ➤ Are employees satisfied with their work?
  - ➤ Are employees satisfied with their salaries?
  - ➤ Do they feel motivated?
  - ➤ Do they feel valued?
  - ➤ Are they loyal to the practice?
  - ➤ Do they feel appreciated and part of the team?
  - ➤ Do they trust their management?
- Employees workload
  - ➤ Do they have good working conditions?
  - ➤ Do they work overtime in acceptable limits?
  - ➤ Do they feel competent and well trained for the work they perform?

❖ **Practice operations**
- Workflow and processes

- ➢ Is the workflow fast enough?
- ➢ How can the workflow speed up?
- ➢ How can work processes be split to make them faster?
- ➢ How can cycle times be improved?
- ➢ What new work measures speed up workflow?
- ➢ What equipments are required to speed up workflow?
- ➢ How can work be redistributed among employees to enhance the workflow?
- ➢ Are work processes inefficient?
- ➢ Can a different work layout speed up the workflow?
- Waiting time
  - ➢ Can the waiting time be reduced and how?
  - ➢ Can the client be kept busy while waiting and how?
  - ➢ Can a different appointments schedule reduce the waiting time?
  - ➢ Does the waiting area and reception require changes to speed up client registration?
- Status of equipments and machinery
  - ➢ How old are equipments and machinery?
  - ➢ Are equipments and machinery outdated?
  - ➢ Are equipments and machinery in working condition?
  - ➢ Does staff use equipments and machinery to satisfying extent?
  - ➢ Does the practice need new equipments and machinery?
  - ➢ Is an upgrade of equipments and machinery possible?
  - ➢ Is a different location of equipments and machinery improving their frequency of use?
  - ➢ Is maintenance for equipments and machinery correctly done and on time?
- Introduction of new services
  - ➢ When were new services introduced for the last time?
  - ➢ Are clients requesting new services?
  - ➢ What services can be introduced without large investment?
  - ➢ When will a new service bring return on investment?
- Income and profitability
  - ➢ Are there ways to improve the income?
  - ➢ How can unnecessary costs be reduced?
  - ➢ What measures can be taken to raise profitability?
  - ➢ How can profitability of staff be increased?
- Facilities and premises
  - ➢ Are facilities and premises in good condition?
  - ➢ Are facilities and premises well maintained?
  - ➢ Has the practice sufficient space?
  - ➢ Are facilities and premises matching the current scope of work?
  - ➢ Are facilities and premises in a good location?
  - ➢ Is an expansion of facilities and premises possible?
  - ➢ How much does an expansion of facilities and premises cost?

❖ **Leadership**
- Perception of senior staff
  - ➢ How does the practice owner or manager regard his leadership skills?
  - ➢ What areas of improvement in leadership can be found?
- Perceptions of employees
  - ➢ How do employees regard the practice owner or manager' leadership skills?
  - ➢ What areas of improvement in leadership can be found?

21.2.3. Step 3 to Excellence

After reviewing above-mentioned and further questions, it is time to integrate excellence into the veterinary practice life.

In this stage, the introduction of a client satisfaction survey and employee satisfaction survey is timely, if not already done. Their outcome provides a good insight into the issues concerning clients as well as employees. Whoever finds surveys too strict can use suggestion boxes that have the same approach of gathering information from clients.

Examples for improvements are manifold. With regard to clients, the main area for improvement is the waiting time, as clients do not appreciate waiting or a very long time. This starts with measuring workflow, cycle times and looking at existing work layouts. Thereafter, the results are used to rearrange the workflow and work processes in order to speed up.

An example for excellence in the field of employees is the use of yearly income target. Those goals are set to encourage employees to bring highest performance. As a reward, a bonus is given if the set target has been achieved. The bonus can be in a monetary form like half or one extra salary or through special training courses. This not only motivates employees, but also actively integrates them into the overall performance goals. Therefore, they can contribute to the overall success and feel more appreciated and valuable for the veterinary practice.

Operational changes lead to major improvements and changes to excellent work in a fast and efficient way. It is good to keep in mind that small changes can have a tremendous positive impact. The work is distributed in a more efficient way among employees resulting in multi-tasking staff. Old and outdated equipments and machinery are replaced, and the new one used to their full capacity. Often suppliers take old equipments and machinery back and offer new ones at discounted prices. Another example in operation's management is the use of radiographic equipment. Excellence is the introduction of a digital X-Ray in the veterinary practice. Despite its higher investment costs compared to a conventional X-Ray, the benefits are manifold. They include higher quality of radiographs, faster developing of X-rays, easier image storage in the patients software file as well as reduced developing costs. Customers greatly appreciate the use of digital radiographs as even tiny fissures can be easily detected due to the outstanding quality of digital X-Rays.

The area of leadership needs two different perspectives to cater for excellence. Firstly, the senior management like practice owner, practice manager or head veterinarian have to evaluate their leadership skills themselves, including possible areas of improvement. Secondly, it is important how the other employees regard the leadership skills of the senior management. Often staff has an entirely different perception of leadership skills than the leaders themselves. However, this can only work if the practice atmosphere is open to change, and employees are not afraid to use constructive criticism. Senior management has to be ready for improvement suggestions as nobody is perfect and can always improve further. An atmosphere of arrogant superiority and intimidation will never lead to excellence and deprive everybody of the change to grow professionally and personally.

21.2.4. Step 4 to Excellence

Without the understanding and commitment of the employees, all efforts for excellence will inevitably fail. Excellence cannot be introduced from the top. It has to come from the hearts and minds of all staff.

Veterinary practice management can play a role model for excellence, but the staff members need to embrace the change. People are often very much afraid of change, as they do not know what this change means for them and how it affects their professional life. Therefore, they must be included in the change to excellence journey, as they will feel less scared and threatened if the change is transparent and in steps. Change should never be imposed from the top. It has to grow from the bottom as a small seed will grow into a big strong plant. Moreover, the culture of outperforming one's self has to be established. This means that nobody should rest on his laurels but be determined to outperform himself. It is good to be satisfied with achievements, but it is imperative to understand that there is still so much more to achieve.

This internal urge to outperform is the strongest driver for excellence. Employees need to realize that if they stop at a certain level, their performance will deteriorate very fast. In contrast, ongoing professional and personal improvement lead to major individual benefits like increased knowledge and skills and thus even higher competitiveness in the veterinary market.

21.2.5. Step 5 to Excellence

The last step in the journey to excellence in the veterinary practice is the introduction of a complete set of work plans, personal development plans, internal policies and procedures as well as risk assessments. Once this has been conducted, it is time to continue the way to excellence by proceeding with the certification process, e.g. with ISO and OHSAS certification. Although it requires a lot of work in the beginning, it is definitely worth the efforts.

To undergo the certification process helps the practice to streamline its work processes and reporting system. Moreover, through the certification process, a standardized system is set up that can be easily followed and later improved further.

This enables new employees to fit in the work routine in a much more efficient and faster way. Furthermore, clients will soon understand that the excellent work that has been certified will improve patient care and therefore, benefit them directly.

21.3. Conclusion

Excellence is an already established part of business management in many companies. In contrast, it just makes its entrance slowly in the veterinary world. Excellence in veterinary practices greatly improves patient care and client satisfaction. Although some professional veterinary organizations start to recommend the introduction of quality management procedures in veterinary practices, the concept of quality management and much more excellence is a relatively new idea that is not widespread yet. To easier understand and implement excellence, it is helpful to go gradually. This includes reviewing of the current situation and determining areas of improvement. The more questions are raised in this context, the better the approach to excellence will become. Excellence is not just an improvement in the medical field. It combines all stakeholders, clients and employees, processes, workflow, external influences to a comprehensive and sound framework. The journey to excellence is a long-term commitment of all employees who need to embrace the culture of change and improvement. The ultimate aim is to provide the best possible patients care, to achieve the highest customer and employee satisfaction and to have latest technology and best administrative procedures in place.

References

[1]   FVE (2002). Federation of veterinarians in Europe. Code of good veterinary practice. http://www.fve.org/news/publications/pdf/gvp.pdf(Accessed on August, 14th, 2011).

[2]   Webster Online Dictionary (2011): Webster's 1913 dictionary. Excellence. http://www.webster-dictionary.org/definition/Excellence (Accessed on August 16th, 2011).

INDEX

J

K

L

M

N

O

P

Q

R